Monday Coffee
& Other Stories of Mothering
Children with Special Needs

Edited by Darolyn "Lyn" Jones
and Liz Whiteacre

Monday Coffee and Other Stories of Mothering Children with Special Needs

Edited by Darolyn "Lyn" Jones and Liz Whiteacre

ISBN: 9780984950133

© 2013 INwords Publications, publishing division of Indiana Writers Center.

All Rights Reserved.

INwords Publications

c/o Indiana Writers Center

PO Box 30407

Indianapolis, IN 46230

www.indianawriters.org

Monday Coffee
& Other Stories of Mothering
Children with Special Needs

Edited by Darolyn "Lyn" Jones
and Liz Whiteacre

INwords Publications
Indianapolis, IN

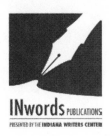

With Support From:

 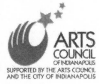 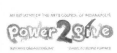 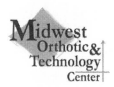

Monday Coffee & Other Stories of Mothering Children with Special Needs

INTRODUCTION

I

II

III

*

Introduction

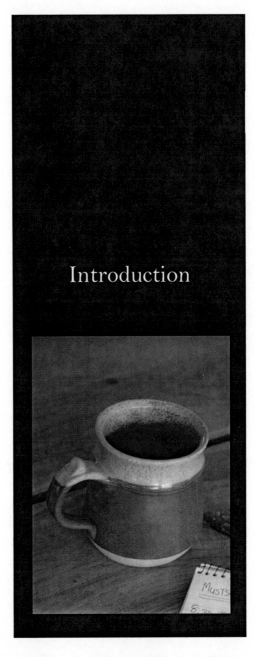

Tell them their child is beautiful, and perfect, and loved. Tell them their child is a profound gift to this world. Because it's all true.

-Heather Kirn Lanier

The Mother's Anthology Project Begins

Liz Whiteacre

When Darolyn Jones walked up with a bright smile after my first English Department meeting at Ball State University, she said, "Hi, I'm Lyn. I've been wanting to talk to you."

A conversation started that day about disability studies, physical therapy, teaching, our families, commuting to Muncie...I later learned that she'd started the Indianapolis Area Special Needs Moms Writing Group and her dissertation stemmed from the writing and relationships she'd developed with those moms. She mentioned the anthology *My Baby Rides the Short Bus: The Unabashedly Human Experience of Raising Kids with Disabilities* (2009), which introduced me to parents writing about parenting their children with special needs. I had spent most of my time consuming writing by disability poets, so I enjoyed this introduction. I asked questions and got to know more about Lyn and her son Will, who has Cerebral Palsy.

Then, I asked to read Lyn's dissertation, *The Joyful Experiences of Mothers of Children with Special Needs: An Autoenthnographic Study.* Though I have not experienced mothering a child who has a disability, I connected with these mothers' stories immediately: I cried, laughed, nodded. In her analysis, Lyn identifies themes that mothers returned to time and again: their challenges, their purpose and providence, and their joy—both simple and pure. There was no pity; anger was explored complexly; and fierce love guided decisions. These women were honest, sometimes painfully, about their motherhood. I was hooked.

"So, what's your plan?" I asked her. "You've got to do something with this."

We made time for coffee in the midst of busy schedules to talk about writing and mothering and realized that through a partnership, we could bring together mothers willing to share their behind-the-scenes stories of raising their children. We put out a call, and amazingly, writers from across the country—and other countries—responded.

The submissions were outstanding, and we used the themes from Lyn's dissertation to guide the selection process and organization of the

i

anthology. What I noticed first, when reading submissions, was that they were about *mothering*. They gave voice to the thoughts that bounced around my head at four in the morning when I pumped breast milk or when I stared at my feverish, three-month-old baby in the hospital as the nurse decided the best place to take a blood sample was a vein in her head. What I realized second was that these mothers couldn't follow along the chapters of the *Academy of American Pediatrics' Caring for Your Baby and Young Child*, which was gifted to me at my shower. They were handed stacks of books (or in some cases, few to none) designed not only to help them navigate mothering their precious babies, but also to help them quickly learn a new language imperative to caring successfully for them. Each was indoctrinated quickly into a high-pressure world of medical-ese, sometimes iffy diagnoses, and scary (often endless) medical procedures—a hazing that did not end when they and their children were released from the delivery room and NICU. Some mothers who submitted had been negotiating this system for over thirty years. As I read, I learned this was high-stakes mothering, day after day, on which the lives of their children depended. And in the midst of my education about these mothers' worlds, I discovered moments to which any parent may relate: the joy they felt snuggling their babies or at their children's first steps, first words; the pride they felt tackling a challenge; the heartache they felt, if they failed to overcome a challenge; or the sorrow of losing their children too soon.

I know Lyn is as thankful as I am to all of the contributing writers, artists, and editors who volunteered to share their stories, talent, and time to make this collection possible. We are very pleased to be published by INwords Press, so that proceeds from this book may return to the Indiana Writers Center's Memoir Project to help fund future projects, which give voice to stories often marginalized. It is our hope that *Monday Coffee & Other Stories of Mothering Children with Special Needs* will inspire you to share your story with us.

Gather or Scatter:
Girlfriending the Special Needs Mom
Darolyn "Lyn" Jones

The Quakers live by an honest creed: "Let your life speak." The message is simple: make sure your life tells the truths you embody.

As an activist, a writer, and mother of a child with special needs, I have adopted this mantra as a way to both make sense of my life and live my beliefs and causes. But, this idea of "speak" connotes a calm and consistent course. And the reality is that sometimes my life is screaming and sometimes it's whispering, but it's always speaking, in fact...it never shuts up.

And I need my girlfriends to listen to it all. I am fortunate to have several girlfriends who have stuck with me for years.

I was the late bloomer in my bunch of girlfriends. I married later, and when I finally became pregnant, most of my married girlfriends were finished having their children. Having a baby meant I could finally catch up and speak this wonderful language they had already been speaking for years.

But as it turned out, I would again remain the outsider. I never got to speak their language because my son suffered a traumatic brain injury in utero, due to a burst blood vessel in my placenta, and lost blood, which is oxygen, which is life. In medical terminology, he was premature, hypoxic, a Hematocrit score of 16, and an Apgar score of 0. Born dead.

I won't go through the other thirty-nine days we spent in the NICU. Or the last ten years of thirty-four procedures or surgeries, thousands of therapies, hundreds of doctor appointments, and more heartache and pure joy than anyone who doesn't live this life can understand. And while the NICU was the biggest battle in this long war torn life I do battle in, others have come much closer. This life of being a mother to a special needs child is the most satisfying, but also the most exhausting.

All mothers redefine their lives and their roles once they have children, but special needs mothers redefine our lives and redefine our lives and redefine our lives because our lives are layered in complexities that at times it seems no one understands or cares about. Our children don't develop typically, therefore, neither do we. Being a special needs mom can be lonely and isolating. It means feeling guilt, sadness, and joy simultaneously. I have had to accept that Will won't walk, won't eat, and won't talk.

When Will entered the living world, my girlfriends either gathered or scattered. In my immediate circle of girlfriends, we had been though many life crises. We knew what to say when someone divorced. We knew what to say when someone had cancer. We knew what to say when someone suffered a miscarriage. But, no one knew what to say when one of us had a child born dead, who if he lived, would face a life of being severely disabled.

Some scattered from the get-go, sending only a card, and not just any card, but a "Congratulations, you had a baby!" card with happy, yellow, pink, and blue baby images. Some gathered at the beginning and scattered later. I knew they would as their gathering was uncomfortable. They would look down at their hands, trying to fill the awkward silence with overly simplistic or unrealistic clichés like:

- "We have a retarded child at our church, and she is very happy." (I found the R-Word offensive before and now even more so.)
- Or, "You can always have another one." (Sure, I'll just replace him. Good plan.)
- And my favorite, "The doctors don't know what they are talking about; he will be fine!" (Glad you feel better saying that, but I don't trust your medical opinion or simple optimism.)

The ones who gathered and stuck with me were the honest ones. They weren't necessarily any more comfortable, but they didn't present me with false hope or clichés. They cried for me and with me. They sat for hours next to Will's bed in the NICU with me. They cleaned my house and cooked meals for me. They weeded my beloved garden when I couldn't.

Several of my very close girlfriends have even had the courage to ask me some difficult questions about how they should or shouldn't respond to me—admitting that sometimes they just don't know what to do or what to say. So, here are my answers:

> • It's okay to ask me how my child is today, but it's not okay to always pair it with a look of pity. I don't want you to

feel sorry for me, but I do want to know you care.

• It's okay to ask me how I am feeling, but know that I may reply with "I'm fine" just because I am tired of always saying I'm not. Ask me specifics. For, example, How have you been sleeping?; How is Will doing with his new pump?; or How are you and Jim handling this recent setback with Will?

• It's okay to ask me to go out—to dinner, to shop, to have coffee. In fact, please include me. Many of the times, I will have to say no because of the demands of Will's care coupled with full time work, but I need to know that you still want me to go out with you. What matters to me is that I am still a part of the group.

• It's okay to complain about your children's problems to me. Your children's problems aren't anything like my child's problems, but they are legitimate to you, and I respect that. Besides, I crave some sense of normalcy, and I want to commiserate with you as you do with me. But, please don't liken your kid's ear infection to Will's five pneumonias that have left him hospitalized and with scarred lungs because they just aren't the same.

• It's okay to talk to me about things you think that I might think are insignificant compared to my world. Picking out a paint color for your living room or rereading a confusing email from a manipulative co-worker is a wonderful diversion for me and helps me know I am still one of the girls.

• It's okay to offer to help me, but mean it and be genuine and honest about what you are and are not willing to do. I probably won't ask for help. We special needs moms rarely ask for help because we often feel like a burden. Offer a task directly. If you are uncomfortable watching Will, then just simply offer to hang out with me for an afternoon while I care for Will. Offer to pick up his medicines at the pharmacy. Offer to come fold the never-ending laundry pile that comes with his involved medical care.

• It's not okay for me to indulge in poor choices or obsess. Tell me I am off base. Don't just think to yourself, *Well, poor Lyn, her life is so hard now—we'll just have to look the other way or ignore it.*

• It's okay to bring the outside world to me. I can't get out as much as I used to. Bring wine, food, and conversation to my house instead.

- It's okay to learn about my world. In fact, come with me to Will's doctor or therapy appointment. Visit Will in the hospital. See my world through me— first hand. Don't see it as a mission trip, but as an opportunity to learn about a new world, learn my language.

- It's okay to make me laugh. My world is often difficult and dark, and I need to laugh. My world is serious, so help me remember there is more than this.

- It's okay to ask me questions about what is or is not okay.

We special needs moms still need our girls. Gather, please.

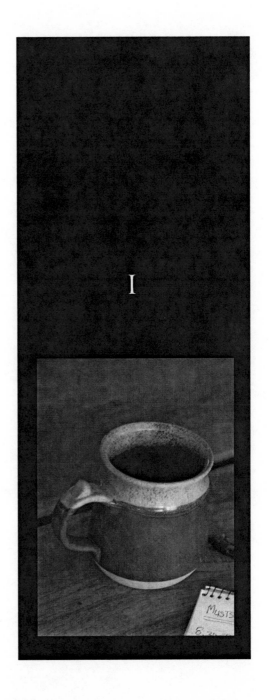

I

I know the only way to deal with this fear is to walk through it —
to feel it, to taste it, to be one with it and to move on.

-Leslie Mahoney

Monday Coffee
Jo Pelishek

Monday. I imagine a quiet morning and a steaming cup of coffee. Karl pulls at the blankets, bringing me back to reality. He was awake until 12:30 a.m., crawled in with us, hogging my pillow the rest of the night. Emily was up several times, calling for Daddy and wanting to be rocked.

A short night, too little sleep and a late start are not the best way to begin a new week. Rick stumbles toward the shower. I attempt to wake the children.

"Karl, time to get up."

"Go away!" he mumbles, pulling the blankets over his head.

Moving to the next room, I expect a better response.

"Erika, Emily, time to get up. It's a new day! What would you like to wear to school?"

Erika dives under the covers. Emily cries, "I want Daddy!" Emily has developmental delays, requires much attention.

Lord, I think, mothering isn't what I'd dreamed.

With much coaxing and a few tears, the children make their way to the kitchen. My husband offers hugs to all and leaves for work.

"I want pancakes," demands Karl.

"Honey, we don't have time for pancakes. How about frozen waffles?"

"No! I want pancakes, pancakes!" He pauses, "OK, give me some toast," he concedes.

"I want waffles," Erika says.

"Waffles, I want waffles too," Karl says, panicking there may not be enough for them both.

Praying, I open the freezer and say a quick thank you. There are enough waffles for two.

I ask Emily what she'd like. Please, not waffles. We're so close to an encounter with contentment.

"I want toast, Mommy!" Yes! There is a God.

"OK, Emmy, toast."

"Mom, I'm having three pieces of toast after my cereal. That's all. Erika, pass the juice," says Mary, our middle schooler. Mary joined our

1

family at age 13, after a history of experiencing abuse and neglect in other settings.

"Syrup, more syrup!" yells Karl, not caring that the syrup is within his grasp.

"You can reach it, honey. I'm making Emily's toast."

"I want Mommy get it," he begins, "Mommy, Mommy get it. Get me syrup!"

Suddenly I remember Karl has not yet had his Attention Deficit Hyperactivity Disorder meds and needs them now! They're prescribed to help control ADHD-like symptoms.

"He's looking at me," whines Erika.

"I want Daddy!" cries Emily.

"Mom, where are my glasses?" asks Mary.

Pounding the table, Karl begins to sing.

Matt, our knowledgeable teenager, strolls through. "What's your problem, Karl? Can't get anything yourself?" Karl responds with a series of shrill squeals. They've played this game before.

It's 7:45 a.m., and we must leave the house by the time the big hand is on the 12.

I quickly crush Karl's pills in the not-so-handy pill crusher. Dutifully, I find two spoons and a carton of ice cream. With some precision, I scoop a small amount onto the first spoon, mold it slightly with my finger, use the second spoon to add just enough ice cream to cover the med without dripping over the edge should this process be delayed.

"Karl," I force a smile, "here's your pill—just how you like it!"

"No, I don't want that stuff! Get it out of my face!"

"Karl," I reply calmly, "Mommy can't put the spoon in your mouth without being close to your face. I need you to cooperate."

"I'm not taking it. It's yucky and I hate it!"

"Please don't yell," I remind him. "You're hurting your vocal chords."

I'm frustrated as I listen to the abuse we've been trying to eliminate through weeks of speech therapy.

The clock is ticking. "Erika, run upstairs and get dressed, OK?"

"I want Mommy to help," she says, defiant as she demands her share of attention in this chaos. Erika is the most capable, independent of the three little ones, but she's determined she'll not be cheated of equal time. It's difficult living with three of four siblings who have a variety of disabilities.

"Karl, please!" I say firmly. "You need to take your med so you can get dressed."

"Mom!" Mary shouts. "I need a picture of a plant for school. Tell Em to quit dancing around, will you?" I hand her a gardening magazine while spotting her glasses on the kitchen sink.

"I'm dressed, Mommy!" announces Emily proudly.

"Yes, sweetheart," I say with a sigh. "You're having a good morning."

"I am too," yells Erika as she places her arms across her chest and sticks out a pouty lip.

"You're having a good morning too, Erika," I pacify, wishing it to be so. "Now, please get dressed!"

She firmly plants her feet. "I want you to help me!"

"Karl, last time! Now open your mouth and take this!"

He lifts his head from his lap. He slaps at the spoon catching me off guard and spilling the contents onto the table. He resumes his hiding position.

"Karl!" I yell, no longer able to restrain my volume. "Enough!"

I attempt to lift his rigid body off the chair. He fights me. "Honey, we need to go!"

He struggles as I try to carry him, falling to his knees on the blue carpet in the living room. For just a moment, I daydream about sitting quietly with a hot cup of flavored coffee and a book. The thought is short-lived.

I give Karl a soft swat on the bottom, place him back on the kitchen chair and scoop the mess from the table. Please Lord, we have to leave!

Karl, eyes puffy, opens his mouth for the med. I notice a bruise appearing on his cheek where he must have bumped it as he fought to keep me at a distance. As I steer him to the bathroom where his clothes are laid out, he complains his knees hurt from having fallen. I make a note of this in his notebook, my communication with his teacher. My heart aches for this little boy with autism, sometimes so uncontrollable and so easily hurt. I open my arms, and we hold each other as he sobs, and I wonder how we can avoid this craziness tomorrow. While Karl protests, I run upstairs to help Erika, picking Emily up on the way.

Mary yells from her room, "I can't get this stupid shoe untied, Mom!"

Erika, her sense of independence returning, refuses my

suggestions for attire but insists I keep her company while she pulls on her blue sweatshirt, black and white striped pants, and purple socks. Wardrobe is near the bottom of the list today. The goal is just to have all of my children wearing clothes.

Trying desperately to be patient I wait for Erika to finish. Meanwhile, I hear Karl pounding on the bathroom door downstairs.

"Karl, you need to get dressed," I yell, wondering whether I, too, will develop vocal nodules from trying to be heard in this not-so-quiet family. I try to remember why we passionately wanted children, worked so hard to have them.

Finally, one by one, the kids are herded to the van. I'll drop them off at school and return home for that quiet cup of coffee. I think I can, I think I can.

"OK, buckle up everybody!" I can almost smell the French vanilla.

"I want to sit in front!"

"You always sit in front!"

"Mom, Matt smiled at me!"

"Where's my seatbelt?"

"Mary, your backpack's in the way. Move over!"

I breathe deeply and silently count. I make my way to the back of the van, reaching to find Karl's seatbelt. As I fish it from the stash of papers and wrappers under the seat, my new watch catches on the upholstery. I add the word "watch" to my mental list of things to get next month. This month's budget is already shot.

While driving and observing the children in the rear view mirror, I wonder how Karl can change so quickly from extreme agitation to calm and quiet. Has the medication taken effect, or does he find the motion of the car soothing? Maybe I should have him get ready for school in the van, as I drive around town.

As I see Karl falling asleep, I'm consumed with panic. In the morning's chaos I'd given him a whole, rather than half a tablet of the new med. Drowsiness is the primary side effect. Rather ironic, I muse, after working so hard to have him take his medication in the first place. I make another notation in Karl's notebook.

After dropping Matt, Mary, and Karl off, each at different schools, I pull into the preschool parking lot. We've logged twenty-two miles, and I'm not home yet. "Do you have your backpacks, girls?"

One look at Emily tells me that she's not feeling well enough for school. I want to cry. She begins to cry. She wants to go. I want her to go. This is supposed to be my time.

Erika hops out of the van. "Goodbye, Mom! I can go by myself. I don't need any help."

"See ya later, Honey."

Emily continues to cry. "My teacher will miss me! I have to go to school."

Oh, I wish you could, Sweetie. I really wish you could. I know how Erika felt earlier. I'm feeling a bit cheated myself. Lord, what about my time?

As we drive toward the too-familiar walk-in clinic, I dream again about coffee. I'm exhausted, and the day has only begun.

After stocking up on Tylenol, antibiotics, and decongestant, Emily and I finally head for home. The answering machine is blinking. Please, Lord, not another sick child.

Karl's teacher has left a message. He's groggy at school, should they skip his noon meds? I call back immediately and hear someone named Shirley at the other end of the line. Wondering why the cook is answering the phone, I explain Karl doesn't need to take his noon meds. I become frustrated—she doesn't understand. I realize that I've called the wrong school.

After snuggling Emily in for a nap and tackling the mounds of laundry, I decide I can sit down with coffee after all. It's 1:30 in the afternoon, and I haven't completed my household tasks. Deep breath. Hot coffee, quiet house. I open my devotional book to today's date. The theme? Strength for the day! Thank you, Lord.

My moments' reverie is interrupted by the telephone. Should I answer? "Hello, Pelishek Zoo. Can I help you?" My friends know when I'm having a bad day.

"Hi, Jodi, it's Kris...the social worker from Karl's school." I wait silently. "I hear you've had a difficult morning. Anything I can do to help?"

She's joking, right? How about a magic medication to improve Karl's behavior? Or a way to help us sleep at night without interruption? Better yet, another miracle, so we don't have these problems at all?

Another miracle. I remember the divine intervention we've already had. Karl was losing touch with reality, and we were advised to place him in an institution. Our little boy, so full of smiles and love, but distant to us then. He has come so far. There's been healing in his life, in our family. Mornings are difficult, but they're only a part of his day. We are all learning, growing. Lord, forgive me.

"It was a crazy morning, Kris, but not unlike most. Just more obvious because of Karl's bruised cheek and my medication error." Is she thinking I am unfit? Could she have heard Karl's shrieks this morning? No. She's concerned, calling to volunteer support.

"I'm going to think of some way to help, Jodi, and when I do, I'll let you know."

You already have, I think, just by calling.

Just then a big yellow bus pulls into our driveway, delivering Erika. Can school be over already? We prepare to repeat this morning's route, in reverse. Cold coffee remains on the table, untouched. Maybe later.

This trip is less tense than the morning's adventure. Emily is rested, Erika is singing, and according to Karl's notebook, he's had a slow but good day. Mary is excited about an upcoming choir concert, and even Matt's happy, highlighting his classes for me. What a great thing, this parenting business. Aren't kids wonderful? I wouldn't want to be doing anything else. The sun's shining—God is faithful.

After unloading the van of kids, backpacks and security blankets, Rick arrives home. Seeing the folded newspaper and coffee cup on the table, he assumes I've had a peaceful day while he was away at work. Someday, I'll tell him about it. Over a hot cup of flavored coffee.

July 19, 2001
Kimberly Escamilla

Dr. Bond's lips are moving,
but her words are shadows.
"DSM, 6 on the spectrum,
ABA, 40 hours, 40k."

I am externally cool,
my default when catastrophe
is gushing like head wound.
I examine Dr. Bond, her smiling children
framed next to her, disturbingly
healthy and pink.

My eyes rest on her grey cashmere dress,
and there, below her knee and clipboard,
a run in her nylons, a slash
all the way to her shiny pumps.

I point it out, almost grinning.

She escorts and leaves me
in the parent self-help corner,
a dumping ground
for the shell-shocked.
Ground zero
for the razed motherheart.

Bite

Kimberly Escamilla

Though men have left their marks
on neck and thigh
and pets have nipped in fear,

nothing could prepare me
for his sealed
mouth on the turn of skin

above my jeans. His teeth
pierced new holes
like into a tongue of leather.

Something feral erected itself
in my raised hand
and swift rap across his head.

The Whole Foods team
offered gauze, gathered
our apples and milk.

No discipline or smile
could erase our scars.
We are canine.

Melting Clocks

Anna Yarrow

"I'll never forget the day my son said he hated me and slammed the door in my face!" My 8-year-old daughter cracks up whenever she hears that voice on the radio: an enthusiastic woman offering to *"Totally transform!"* unruly child behavior.

The first time I heard the ad, alone in my Jeep, I gripped the steering wheel, and snorted bitterly—because *that was my life, every day.* I didn't call the 1-800 number. Didn't buy the program. But I did start to question our *Scary Movie* version of existence. The bites and kicks and scratches that caused me to fear my daughter. Her preference for animals, over humans. Mystery terrors—blue tiles, fluorescent lights, mannequins in a shop window, violin music—sent her into fits—falling to the ground with primal screams, eyes vacant—or running…running *away* from me, across a busy parking lot, into the street, in front of a bus. Bald patches dotted her scalp like crop circles. Before leaving for school each morning, she pulled her socks and shoes on-and-off, on-and-off five times, ten times, I-don't-know-how-many times, and begged to be naked. "You don't love me, because you make me wear clothes!"

Why didn't I seek help sooner? (Actually, I did. But with a squeak, a whisper, that no one heard.) Why is it so hard to write about this? To remove my veil of confusion and shame? To accurately portray my daughter, 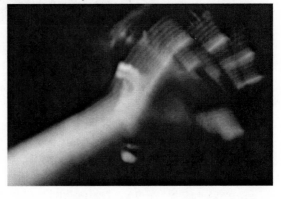 bangs hanging down over her triple-espresso eyes; her genius IQ; her allegiance to riddles and palindromes and optical illusions; her desire to invent new worlds—without hair or loud noises—via magical superpower ice cream?

In Heather Sellers' book, *You Don't Look Like Anyone I Know,* she recalls the time an animal was trapped in her childhood bedroom. From the hallway, she heard it yowl and thump. A cat? Raccoon? Squirrel?

Her schizophrenic mother wouldn't allow her to open the door or go find help, saying, "I just can't deal with it." So they stopped using that room. Ignored the skittering turned dead silence.

When I was growing up, a devil lived in my mom and step-dad's bedroom, orchestrating a bizarre cacophony of sobs and pummels, lamp smashing, wood cracking. For a decade, I tried to shelter my four younger siblings from the evil behind that door. We watched the clock, AM to PM to AM to PM, wondering how long this fighting binge would last. We listened for the swivel-click of the doorknob—signal of our zombie parents emerging.

What is love?

What is normal?

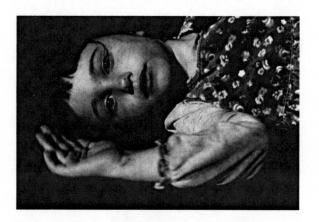

Teachers praised my daughter: "She reads 100 books a week!" "She finishes her worksheet before the other kids have even written their names at the top of the page." "She's brilliant." "Confident." "Quirky."

But I felt the absence of reciprocal love and saw that she had no friends. Instead of playing, she spent recess in the class potato patch, digging up tubers and muttering to herself. She had frequent tantrums and visits to the principal's office.

I was a single Mom, working nine to five at a minimum wage job to provide for us. After school, she went by van to an all-girl daycare. Sometimes the driver phoned me in exasperation, saying, "Your daughter won't get on the van" or "Your daughter won't get *off* the van!" One day, she collapsed on the pavement, saying, "My legs won't move! I can't go in there!" I heard the teachers' pleading and her refusal—a frenetic dirge, like whale song, whipping my soul. At pick-up time, she avoided my eyes. "You don't listen to me! You don't understand me!" Every night an argument. A fury.

Desperate for help, I requested assessment through the Santa Fe Public School system. Specialists conducted tests, over winter, spring, and summer and finally diagnosed her, at age seven, with High Functioning Autism, also called Asperger's Syndrome. In the fall, they formed a support team of therapists and enrolled her in gifted and special ed. classes. I read piles of books about autism and Asperger's, my "Aha!" growing with every word. I put her on a gluten/dairy free diet and added probiotics and vitamins. Her runny nose and digestive problems cleared up. Her defiance abated.

In December 2012, a young man with Asperger's shot and killed 26 people at Sandy Hook Elementary in Connecticut. That same week, during a holiday party at school hosted by a substitute teacher, my daughter threatened to kill herself, after her favorite boy announced, "I'm not going to be your friend!"

Protocol required that I rush her to a state psychiatrist for evaluation. He was teddy-bearish and kind, and she answered his questions with bubbly repartee, explaining, "The party was too noisy and crazy, and I didn't know the lady...I thought it would be much more peaceful to be dead in a hole in the ground...and I've heard heaven is a nice place."

She inspected the artwork on his walls. "Who painted this? I like Picasso and Salvador Dali—especially the melting clocks."

They debated, and she refused to sign an affidavit, which read, *I promise not to harm myself.* Reasoning, "I don't *know* what will happen in the future. Right now I'm fine. But sometimes I get upset, and it feels like I'm exploding."

He chuckled and said, "She's only in second grade? Quite a kid!"

What is it like to be the mother of a child with special needs? You feel inadequate. Perplexed. You feel like crying, as if you're swimming in a subterranean bog of sorrow. You implode and howl silently.

My daughter has only seen me cry once. (An event she recalls fondly, saying, "Hey Mom, remember that time you cried?") A bad day, long ago, when PMS and bills and an Asper-girl felt like too much to handle. I sat cross-legged in the middle of her giraffe-print rug and let my tears fall. I pointed to my cheeks and said, "Look! I'm crying!"

She glanced at me for a brief second, and murmured, "That's not real!"

She tugged the navy blue comforter off her bed and threw it over my head, tucking it around my body. Then she tiptoed out and shut the door.

At a Quaker meeting, I heard a spritely octogenarian woman tell her life story. Born to missionary parents in China. Political rallies. A college romance. Marriage. And, "Then I raised four kids." Earned a graduate degree. Wrote a book. Wait...did she say—*then I raised four kids?* All the labor of motherhood, condensed into one sentence.

Before the diagnosis, my daughter and I traveled through months of bad days. But now, the bad days have shrunk to bad hours or only minutes. She's learned how to self-regulate, to calm herself, to express her feelings appropriately. To say, "I'm sorry."

She expresses empathy, like "I saw a man in a wheelchair. I'm sad he can't walk." Therapy has taught her to recognize faces and emotions. "Mom? Are you *angry?* Your eyes are wide, and you're talking loud."

She walks into the room and peers at the computer screen. "Are you writing about me again, Mom? You know, you've got to consider my reputation. Will people like me, when they meet me? You've got to write lots of good things, too. You should write about animals."

I ask her to recite a poem for me. Something funny. She blushes and jumps on my bed.

"Ok."

There is the terrible 20 ft Feezus. Shhhhh. I don't think he sees us!
This is the tail of the man-eating Fullet. Let's not pull it!

She runs to find a Shell Silverstein tome on the shelf and insists on reading forty-three poems aloud, before brushing her teeth.

"Write about the hamster, Mom. Write about the cats!"

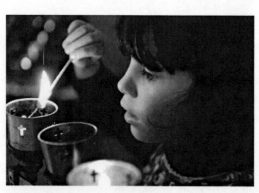

When our hamster died, my daughter said, "Let's put it outside to decompose."

Our cats used to hide behind the couch, to elude the girl-child's rough hugs and high-pitched, "I love you I love you!" Accompanied by near strangulation. But now, they approach her and settle into her lap for gentle snuggles. She strokes their calico fur and sings, "You are beautiful kitties." Her songs spiral up the staircase and sway the cobwebs in the rafters.

She's making friends: kids who frolic with her in the hot tub and play doodle games on the iPad. We have a new home, with deer camping in our backyard, and a fox that visits each night. I work part time, so I can pick her up from school.

The bell rings at three o'clock. Children stream through the doorways, toting backpacks and science projects. Daffodils and tulips jive in spring. I scan the crowd, until suddenly, one dazzling girl chooses me with her eyes, and I beam and choose her too. We race towards each other, and I clasp her small hand in mine.

Resources

Ashley, Susan. *The Asperger's Answer Book: The Top 275 Questions Parents Ask.* USA: Sourcebooks, Inc., 2006. Print.

Attwood, Tony. *The Complete Guide to Asperger's Syndrome.* USA: Jessica Kingsley Pub., 1754. Print.

Attwood, Tony, Temple Grandin, Tresa Bolick, Catherine Faherty, Lisa Iland, Jennifer McIlwee Myers, Ruth Snyder, Shelia Wagner, and Mary Wrobel, *Asperger's and Girls.* USA: Future Horizons, 2006. Print.

Bock, Kenneth and Cameron Stauth. Healing the New Childhood Epidemics: Autism, ADHD, Asthma, and Allergies: The Groundbreaking Program for the 4-A Disorders. USA: Ballantine Books, 2008. Print.

Grandin, Temple. *Different . . . Not Less.* USA: Future Horizons, 2012. Print.

Isaacson, Rupert. *The Horse Boy: A Father's Quest to Heal His Son.* USA: Little, Brown and Company, 2009. Print.

Lovecky, Deirdre. *Different Minds.* USA: Jessica Kingsley Pub., 2003. Print.

McCandless, Jaquelyn, Jack Zimmerman, and Teresa Binstock. *Children With Starving Brains: A Medical Treatment Guide for Autism Spectrum Disorder.* USA: Bramble Books, 2009. Print.

Robison, John Elder. *Look Me In The Eye: My Life with Asperger's.* USA: Three Rivers Press, 2008. Print.

Sellers, Heather. *You Don't Look Like Anyone I Know.* USA: Riverhead Trade, 2011. Print.

Silverstein, Shell. *Don't Bump the Glump!: and Other Fantasies.* 2nd edition. USA: HarperCollins, 2008. Print.

Stagliano, Kim. *All I Can Handle: I'm No Mother Teresa: A Life Raising Three Daughters with Autism.* USA: Skyhorse Publishing, 2011. Print.

Verdick, Elizabeth and Elizabeth Reeve. *The Survival Guide for Kids with Autism Spectrum Disorders (And Their Parents).* USA: Free Spirit Publishing, 2012. Print.

Yanofsky, Joel. *Bad Animals: A Father's Accidental Education in Autism.* USA: Arcade Publishing, 2012. Print.

The Caves of Chattanooga
Suzanne Kamata

"There's always one more cave to explore."
–Johnny Cash, "Another Song to Sing"

When I tell Lilia that we are going to view bats, she is scared at first. She knows bats only from horror movies and vampire stories in her favorite manga. All the same, she is willing to go. My concerns, as usual, are about accessibility.

We are in the Southeast on our first mother-daughter trip. My husband and son are back home in Japan, busy with work, summer school, and baseball practice. My thirteen-year-old daughter Lilia and I won't be on our own, however. We've made plans to travel to Tennessee with my extended family.

I hadn't known what we would do in Chattanooga. I'd left everything up to my sister-in-law who first suggested the trip as an alternative to a few days at the beach. Although I love the coast of South Carolina—the salt marshes, the frolicking dolphins, the sweetgrass basket sellers on the side of the road—I conceded that it was too hot to think about sitting by the ocean. I could imagine the white sand searing the soles of our feet, the sun burning our necks and shoulders. It has been one of the hottest summers on record, with the mercury topping the hundred degree mark for days in a row. The mountains of Tennessee will be cooler, I think. Plus, my fourteen-year-old nephew, an avid runner who's been on the varsity cross-country team since middle school, wants to run on a particular mountain trail in Chattanooga. Our destination was decided.

I've been to Chattanooga once before, as a child. I remember being on top of Lookout Mountain, peering down from dizzying heights, at rocks and trees below. I recall reports of Japanese tourists who've fallen into the Grand Canyon while trying to get the perfect snapshot, and I have a horrible image of my daughter's wheelchair going over a rocky cliff. I hope there are guardrails along the mountain trails—tall ones. I also have a memory of garden gnomes in fairy tale settings, something that I'm sure my daughter would enjoy.

I entrust my sister-in-law with the hotel reservations. I don't mention that we need a handicap accessible room. My sister-in-law knows that Lilia can't walk and that she will need her wheelchair. Surely, she doesn't need to be reminded, although come to think of it, my husband rarely thinks to mention our special needs when making reservations. On our last trip—to Tokyo Disneyland—we had to carry Lilia up the stairs to our second-floor motel room.

I also remember numerous play dates with mothers of able-bodied kids who promised to help get my daughter's wheelchair up hills and staircases, to help my daughter navigate complicated jungle gyms and climbing structures. "Helping" always turned out to be more arduous than others expected, and more often than not, I was the only one helping my daughter up ladders, through tunnels, and down slides while my well-meaning-but-oblivious mommy friends chatted on park benches.

But then my parents, who are also going on the trip, assure me that my sister-in-law is working on getting an accessible room. Well, that's one thing I don't need to worry about.

Chattanooga, a town of brick and crepe myrtle backed by hazy mountains, is about a six-hour drive from Lexington, South Carolina, our starting point. It takes us a little longer to get there because we make a couple of pit stops—one, at a McDonald's where I find that the toilet paper and soap dispensers in the "accessible" bathroom are too high for a wheelchair user to reach.

Lilia occupies herself with a thick manga and a DVD with Japanese subtitles that we brought along as we cruise down Bobby Jones Highway past trees and trees and trees. About the only things of interest for many miles are the sign indicating the exit for the Laurel and Hardy Museum, and a couple of fawns lazing by the side of the road.

In early afternoon, we arrive at the hotel and convene with my brother and his family. Lilia, who in addition to having cerebral palsy is deaf, manages to converse with her cousins through flashcards that she made in advance and Google translate. (Thank goodness for Wifi!)

My brother has scouted out a cave from which we can watch bats emerge at dusk. We've made plans to check it out the following evening.

Nickajack Cave was once a refuge for Native Americans and a hideout for pirates who preyed on travelers who came down the Tennessee River. Later, during the Civil War, it was mined for saltpeter, which is used to make gunpowder. At one time, the cave was even used as a dancehall, and it has been immortalized in song on more than one occasion. A suicidal Johnny Cash allegedly came up with the words for "Another Song to Sing" inside the cave. YouTube also turned up the tune "Nickajack Cave," by singer-songwriter Kevin Bilchuk, which is about how Cash found redemption while crawling around on his hands and knees in the cavern. In 1967, the cave was partially flooded after the construction of Nickajack Dam and is now a sanctuary and maternity roost for the endangered gray bat.

We park at the Maple View Recreation Area, near the edge of the reservoir. Luckily, there is a boardwalk leading through trees to the bat-viewing platform. My brother and niece are already waiting when Lilia and I arrive with my parents. My sister-in-law and nephew have gone for a run around the reservoir. We can see their small shapes across the water.

It's about an hour till dusk, but already another group of three has staked out a spot on the platform: a young pony-tailed woman sporting a pink T-shirt, shorts, and a nose-ring; another young woman with glasses sitting on the railing; and a bearded guy with a long-lensed camera. The young woman with glasses is holding a net, and Lilia wonders in sign language if it's for catching bats.

The woman laughs when I inquire about the net. "No, it's for catching insects." Her sister, the woman with the nose ring, is a PhD candidate at the University of Tennessee in the study of bats. She already has a Master's degree from the University of Hawaii, where, she informs us, there is only one indigenous species, *lasiurus cinereus*, otherwise known as the hoary bat.

We can see that the cave is cordoned off, and a sign juts from the water at the entrance, declaring it off-limits to human visitors. This, the bat scholar informs us, is to prevent the spread of white-nose syndrome, a disease that threatens the bat population. Once a colony is infected, the disease spreads quickly and has killed at least ninety-five percent of bats at some locations in only two years.

As dusk gathers, fireflies spark in the trees. Mosquitoes alight on my bare legs. I want the bats to come and eat the bugs. My sister-in-law and nephew return from their run. A family from Chicago joins us on the platform, and then a couple of guys and a dog in a boat pull up in front of the cave, the sound of the outboard motor disrupting our peaceful interlude. Their loud voices, twanged with Tennessee accents, blare across the water. "C'mon bats," one guy yells impatiently. Like us, they are here to see the gray bats emerge from the cave, but they are hardly respectful. They go beyond the sign, into the mouth of the cave, before anchoring just outside and diving into the water.

The PhD student is horrified. She has explained earlier, about the special Tencel suits that students wear when entering bat caves, the extraordinary measures to which they go in order to prevent the spread of disease. "I hope they get rabies," she snarls.

One of the guys swims to shore and climbs up the embankment, then jumps ten feet from the cliff, splashing into the water below.

We wonder out loud if this is disturbing the bats.

Meanwhile, Lilia keeps asking me what people are talking about. She doesn't quite get this American custom of speaking to strangers. She thinks that we must all know each other. I try to keep her in the flow—now we're wondering if there is poison ivy in these woods; now we're talking about how those guys in the boat weren't supposed to go near the bats; now we're talking about how a scuba diver in pursuit of a giant catfish illegally entered and got lost in Nickajack Cave for 17 hours 20 years ago and how the cave had to be drained. (The diver, David Gant, thought that his rescuers were angels and became a born-again Christian after the event, which became known as "The Bat Cave Miracle.")

Finally, there is a speck overhead, and I point to the darkening sky. The bats have begun to swoop and flutter above the cave. First, just a few, then there are a hundreds of them, a swirl of dark wings. They come diving for insects just above our heads, and then flap again into the treetops. Every night, between April and September, they feast upon thousands of beetles and moths and aquatic insects, devouring up to 274,000 pounds of bugs.

Lilia gazes in wonder at the bats, the fireflies, the stars in the night sky. When we go back to the car, the boardwalk is completely dark. We need a flashlight to find our way. It's too dark to sign in the car, but later, Lilia writes in her notebook: "Don't go in the cave! Bats! If you touch leaves, you will be itchy!" She also writes about the man who went into the cave twenty years ago and couldn't find his way back out.

The following morning, as we begin to drive up to the top of Lookout Mountain, my dad recalls how terrified Grandma had been on our first trip here, over forty years ago. Back then, there had been nothing to prevent our freefall should my dad miss a hairpin curve. Things are different now. There are guardrails. The road is wider. There's even a Starbuck's at the summit, across from the entrance to

Rock City Gardens, one of Chattanooga's premier tourist attractions, and home to the garden gnomes I remember from my youth.

According to *The Enchanted Gazette* ("Gnome News is Good News!"), a tourist brochure in the guise of a newspaper, Lookout Mountain, formerly inhabited by Native Americans and site of a major Civil War battle, was first commercialized in 1924 by businessman Garnet Carter, who established the Tom Thumb Golf, the first ever miniature golf course, on top of the mountain. He was also responsible for Fairyland, a residential community inspired by his wife Frieda's interest in European folklore. That explains the gnomes.

There's a ramp at the entrance—so far, so good—but we quickly come upon steps. Our group has scattered by now and my wheelchair bearer brother is nowhere in sight. A Rock City employee tells us that to get to the Mother Goose Village, we'll need to go through a back entrance. We start by exploring the rest of the site.

There's a wide, sloped path going past various flowers and herbs. Lilia likes to take advantage of inclines and coast, whenever possible, but I hang on to the handles of her wheelchair. It's a good thing that I do, because I discover that the end of the path drops off into a crevice.

One path, "Fat Man's Squeeze," is too narrow for the wheelchair, so we have to turn back around. We can't figure out how to get to the Swinging Bridge or the Opera Box Overview, but we do manage to get Lilia to Lover's Leap, from which we can view seven states.

Feeling a bit frustrated, I decide to give up on the more inaccessible areas, and take Lilia to the Fairyland Cavern, a cave full of illuminated dioramas featuring scenes from Cinderella, Hansel and Gretel, and other well-known fairytales. As a child, I found this cave delightful. As an adult, I can't help thinking that it's a bit cheesy, but Lilia, who has been born and raised in the land of Hello Kitty, loves it without a trace of irony, and snaps photos of every display. At the very least, the dark, damp cave offers respite from the summer heat.

We stop by a barbecue joint for lunch before hitting up our next cave on Raccoon Mountain, which according to the tourist brochure I picked up at a rest stop, is "rated number one in the South," with more formations than any other cavern in the region.

"Is it accessible?" I asked my brother earlier.

He told me that he'd called to inquire. "They said there are one hundred steps inside, but no more than ten at a time."

One hundred steps?

He assures me that he will help carry Lilia.

I'm feeling a bit dubious, but I figure that if Lilia can make it up three flights of stairs at school every day by hanging on to the railing, she can probably drag herself up these steps, too. So what if she slows down the guided tour? And if my brother wants to volunteer to carry her wheelchair, then fine. Maybe my able-bodied, fourteen-year-old nephew will pitch in, as well.

We've already purchased our non-refundable tickets online via my brother's smart phone. We pass by a group of muddy-kneed spelunkers, just back from a guided wild cave tour, and go into the gift shop/reception area. The young guy at the cash register insists that we need a print out of our reservation, and that the cave is not wheelchair accessible.

"But we called in advance…" my brother protests.

No matter. Whoever talked to my brother must not know the cave well. We can't take the wheelchair into the caverns. And our tickets are *non-refundable*.

My first impulse is to launch into a rant. *What do you mean this place is inaccessible? My daughter has a right to go into that cave and behold its natural wonders! You are discriminating against us! If Mammoth Cave can admit wheelchair users, then so can you! What about the Americans with Disabilities Act? And what do you mean our tickets are non-refundable?*

However, I don't want to ruin this family outing by making a scene, and we're already holding up the tour group, imposing on strangers. When the manager offers to allow us access to the first cavern and give us credit in the gift shop in exchange for our tickets, I'm willing to compromise. We have forced the staff to confront our situation. Maybe that's a start. Maybe they will consider ways to make the cave more accessible to wheelchair users in the future.

I would like for Lilia to be able to see the stalagmites and stalactites, the rimstone pools and flowstone, the so-named Crystal Palace and Hall of Dreams. I would like for her to feel the spray of the underground waterfall on her face and to be able to cross the natural rock bridges formed by centuries of mineral deposits deep inside. But when I imagine the additional construction that would be necessary to make this cave fully accessible—the concrete and drills and saws—I'm not so sure it's a good idea. Maybe not everyone should go into this wild place, especially if it would mean desecrating its natural beauty. Maybe like Nickajack Cave, we should let it be, a pure place of mystery. Maybe there are some places that Lilia in her wheelchair, and me with her, can do without visiting.

I urge my parents and my brother and his family to go ahead into the cave. Lilia and I wait for our guide, a lanky young man who takes us into the empty first cavern and shines a flashlight on rock striated like bacon, and a cave-dwelling salamander while giving us the official spiel. It's Lilia's first time in such a cave. She likes the sparkle of the quartz, the blue of the salamander. We learn that this dark place is home to a blind species of spider, and also to bats. She takes pictures of various rock formations—a straw, a stalagmite. Our guide lets Lilia hold the flashlight and explore as much as she likes, as long as we don't touch the cave walls. The oil from human skin can hinder the natural flow of water and mineral deposits. When my daughter is satisfied, we go back out into the gift shop, into the light.

Lilia goes straight for the stuffed animals on display and picks up a plush gray bat. I discover that, as in the case of Johnny Cash and David Gant, our evening at Nickajack Cave has made something of a convert out of my daughter. Instead of being chiroptophobic, my daughter is now a bat fan. We get a T-shirt for her brother and the stuffed gray bat to commemorate our trip.

When we are back in Japan, and she begins to tell about our trip, the caves are the first thing that she mentions. She tells how gray bats flew in a funnel up to the sky, how she saw seven states and scenes from fairytales, and how the stone in Raccoon Mountain Caverns sparkled. "*Kira kira,*" she signs, her fingers wiggling in the air.

Manneken Pis
Kimberly Escamilla

It was in the neighborhood of hubris
where you stood atop the slide for the thousandth time.

Maybe you were at war
with the whiny girls in their Baby Lulu frocks.

Perhaps you were lost
in the curve's glimmer like a banana slug in the rain.

Or were you dousing the fire
of tedium between us, weary of my iPod and tea.

A rivulet came before the yelps
and rush of nannies, then it flowed calmly

like the river Senne
wending its way to a pool of sand.

You flew down with the final swell
beaming, wet, heroic.

*Manneken Pis (The Boy Peeing statue in Brussels, Belgium)

Checking on Dinner

Kimberly Escamilla

Today, he was escorted home by a cop.
A couple driving down Hwy 1 saw him
riding his bike into oncoming traffic.
He couldn't say his name.
He was flapping and barefoot.
He was five miles from home and lost for an hour.
I thought he would be at the beach,
I thought he would go to the trees.
Up and down the trail,
I stopped every jogger, "Have you seen…"
The backyard was littered
with silence and overripe plums.
I will never know my son.
Never know which road or cliff is next.
I used to worry that I would kill him.
Now I see that he'll dare the world to.

This House
Linda Davis

Windows

> "The Past is a Window into the Soul
> The Future is a Mirror without any Glass in it."
> —Xavier Forneret

My whole life I've been lucky. When I was twelve, my friends and I entered a writing/drawing contest with a major department store in Boston. There were over 5000 entries. I was one of ten who won. My picture was in all the local papers, and a poster size photo of my likeness hung in the downtown Boston store for over a year.

I've had "born" luck, easily attaining personal goals: becoming a member of the National Honor Society and captain of the track team in high school. And, I've had "superficial" luck: receiving six invitations to the senior prom, winning a radio contest for picking my ten favorite songs, or scoring a single third row ticket for the sold-out Elvis Costello show, just by asking.

A childhood friend once remarked, "You are crazy lucky," after I won an all-school raffle. As I sat ticking off each number that was called out, I thought, *Someone has to win. Why not me?*

My mother once saw a fortuneteller who confirmed my good luck by telling her, "I see a crown on her head, symbolic of incredible happiness."

The one time I saw a fortuneteller, she said, "I've never seen anything like this. Such good luck! Please come back in ten years and tell me all that's happened to you."

My lucky streak continued into my twenties and thirties where I successfully landed great jobs for *Harper's Magazine* in New York and Robert Redford's production company in Los Angeles.

In my late thirties, I married my husband George. We conceived on our honeymoon, which given the number of miscarriages and fertility treatments all of our thirty-five+ aged friends were going through, seemed lucky too. I went into labor on my birthday, and even though Noel was born the day after my birthday, I considered it the ultimate cosmic birthday gift to have a child born so close to me.

Unlike many Los Angeles transplants, I had the good fortune of having my mother move to Los Angeles. As other transplants with children know, having family nearby is a saving grace.

A month after we had Noel, we bought an old house, which we renovated. Six months later, the real estate market shifted dramatically. Two years later, it was worth twice what we paid for it. More luck.

Two years after Noel was born, we conceived a second son within a month of trying. Again, the fertility Gods were smiling on us.

Even my bad luck was somehow good. One rainy night, back when I lived in Boston, a car crashed into mine on the i-95 freeway, setting fire to my car and trapping me in on the driver's side by the median. I got myself out seconds before the car blew up. What did all the firemen say when they arrived?

"Ma'am, do you have any idea how lucky you are?!"

It's true I've had my share of disappointments and setbacks: alcoholic father, parents who were too wrapped up in divorce to help me make good choices about my future, and open heart surgery for my mother, to name a few. But while my bad luck could be described as typical, my good luck was decidedly not.

Floors

"Circumstances are like clouds, continually gathering and bursting. While we are laughing, the seed of some trouble is put into the wide arable land of events. While we are laughing, it sprouts, it grows and suddenly bears a poison fruit we must pluck."

–John Keats

When Noel was two and a half years old and Julian was eight months, I was strolling with them in front of Santa Monica's City Hall. Noel began to rub his hands together in a quick, repetitive motion. He'd been doing this for about a week. George and my mother thought it was cute; that he was imitating his baby brother Julian. It troubled me.

As I leaned forward to maneuver the double stroller up a steep curb, the word "autism" suddenly came into my head. I had zero knowledge of what autism was other than having seen the movie "Rainman." Yet, like my certainty that I, as much as anyone, had a chance of winning the school raffle, somewhere in my mind I already knew this word was relevant to my life.

When I got home, I quickly ran to get my *What to Expect: The Toddler Years* book; the same one I'd consulted for sleeping, feeding and other developmental hurdles, which at the time seemed insurmountable. I looked up autism in the glossary and found the page in the book. There were ten bullet points listing the characteristics of children with autism. Noel answered to eight of them. The description of autism read:

> Autism is a syndrome characterized by impairments in social relatedness, language and communication, a need for routine and sameness, abnormal movements and sensory dysfunction. Autism is a lifelong condition. (Eisenberg and Murkoff 713)

I lay face down on the floor in my bedroom, unable to move for a long time, inhaling carpet when I was inhaling at all. Noel and Julian were in the bath at the time and soon began calling to me. It took tremendous effort for me to go to them because I didn't want to see Noel in a different way. It was two hours before George would arrive home from work. I couldn't tell him over the phone. That much I knew. I desperately wanted to sleep, certain that if I could only lose consciousness I would wake up and discover this had never happened.

After I toweled the children off, I put them under the covers of our bed, hoping to lose myself in the folds of the covers—a compromise to sleep. I remember feeling like I was looking down at us from overhead and seeing an X-ray of our bodies: Noel with a broken brain, me with a broken heart. The phone rang. I knew it was George. He always called around this time. I thought about not answering, but selfishly I wanted to hear his voice, even if I couldn't tell him. Maybe it would help comfort me. Didn't work. His first question, as always was, "How are the boys?"

"Good," I said without a second's hesitation.

I quickly got off the phone, using Julian as an excuse. As I hung up, I remember envying George's last two hours of ignorance of Noel's condition. Two hours later, when I showed him the book, he fell to the floor and, unlike me, wept profusely.

The next day, we paid an emergency visit to Noel's pediatrician, Dr. W. After observing Noel for over a half-hour, he declared, "I'd be very surprised if this was anything neurological." As much as I wanted desperately to believe him, I knew he was wrong.

Even with his misgivings, Dr. W. referred us to neurologist, Dr. C, whom we had to wait an agonizing forty-eight hours to get in to see. Finally, we made our way to her cluttered windowless office, ominously located just above a children's cancer clinic. Dr. C. did not smile or attempt to ease the burden of bad news with any smiles or consolatory remarks. She diagnosed Noel as autistic as casually as if she'd told us he had a minor cold. It took five minutes.

You may be wondering why no one had noticed Noel's autism sooner? I'll try to explain. Noel was our firstborn. Although I'd done more than my share of babysitting through the years, this was my first experience with a baby. So, I relied on professionals. He'd been at nursery school and seen by various healthcare professionals his whole life (when he was one, he had a blocked tear duct that required a minor operation). Although he'd walked late, many children do, and as long as he did by eighteen months, Dr. W. wasn't concerned. While he didn't demonstrate any interest in his peers, Noel was intensely focused on adults, especially those closest to him. He certainly had no aversion to being touched. If anything, he sought it out, burrowing under covers and pillows and reaching his small hands to fit inside my shirtsleeves. (Later, we would discover that this was indicative of sensory issues: a component of autism.) He also had language. Language plays a crucial role in autism. It's the yardstick by which many children are measured: those who talk and those who don't. Noel spoke from the time he was eight months old, sooner than his typically developing brother, although, at age two, when Noel should have progressed to full sentences, he was still stuck on single words. Lastly, we had the example of Dr. W. stating his disbelief at Noel's diagnosis. So, instead of being hard on myself for not knowing sooner that Noel was autistic, I opted for my last sliver of confidence-building in the dreary, hopeless shattered dream days after Noel's diagnosis: I had been the one who had diagnosed him. Dr. Temple Grandin, the most famous, well-educated autistic person in the world who has garnered national attention for her award-winning designs of humane slaughterhouses says early diagnosis is tantamount to progress. Ironically, perhaps this had been, my last dance with good fortune: diagnosing my own son's tragic misfortune. Needless to say, we never went back to Dr. W. again.

In the past, whenever I'd felt scared or received bad news I would think/wish/pray my way out of it. Things I couldn't change—my mother's bad heart, or my own broken heart—fixed themselves with time. When Noel was diagnosed, I remember thinking initially that I could outsmart fate, as I always had.

This time, there was no out.

A dear friend said to me, "We're at an age when we'll all receive our share of bad luck: diseases, death, tragedy. This is yours." My good luck had come to a halting conclusion.

Nails

"There is nothing so much as gratifies an ill tongue as when it finds an angry heart."

–Thomas Fuller

Most of what I remember of Noel's first being diagnosed is not about Noel, but rather, George and me. A psychologist we saw told us, "The attrition rate of marriages among parents with children on the autistic spectrum is incredibly high." It's easy to see why. Well-punctured hearts seem intent on adding more nails. There are the thoughts you share, like being hypersensitive to each other's short-comings with regards to caretaking, and the thoughts you don't share, the ones where you blame each other's genes for your child's diagnosis.

Granted, we had some help here. When a child is diagnosed with autism, parents bring their child to a series of professionals who require them to fill out personal questionnaires the size of novellas. Sample questions include everything from: "Describe your pregnancy in detail," to "Do you have any relatives with odd social behaviors?" While the former question is obvious, the latter seems less so, until the fifth or sixth time you answer it. Thus begins an internal quest to nail the genealogical source of your child's affliction, which inevitably lands on your partner's family tree. Sure, I had an odd aunt that never married and didn't talk to my parents for years at a time because she held a grudge over some inconsequential event. And then there was the time my father casually mentioned in conversation that sometimes he would cross over to the other side of the street to avoid running into an acquaintance. But for the most part, these minor citations paled in comparison to George's cast of odd relatives, including all those I'd never met who lived in England. Everyone knows England is the world's unofficial capital for human eccentricity.

After a while, I began to want to blame more tangible things than in-laws I'd never met. No aspect of our lives was removed from this intense scrutiny. It's impossible to guess how many hours I have spent in an internal investigation of what caused Noel's autism. Was it the diluted margarita I had when I was breastfeeding? The time he fell off the bed and hit his head on a sharp corner of the wall? Maybe there's something in our drinking water? The ocean water? The multiple vaccines laced with mercury? Something he contracted on our trip to Mexico? The drugs from the root canal I had a month after he was delivered that he too would get via breastfeeding? The unruly collection of electrical wires that sits off to the right side of our house? The light mold that sometimes surfaces on the ceiling, just above Noel's bed? The multiple jars of peanut butter I consumed when pregnant? George's saccharine intake? The cats' dander? A toxic flower in our garden? Los Angeles? Boston? Every place in between?

My preoccupation eventually led me to a theory that wasn't scientific, but rather, superstitious. I was tricked. Two and a half years of having a healthy baby was a lie. The smiling faces in Noel's baby books? Lies. The baby shower and gifts of best wishes? Lies. The heartfelt toasts at our wedding? Lies. Our engagement and three+ years of carefree dating? Lies. In fact, my whole life of good luck had been a lie. It was all a set-up for what happened with Noel. The Gods were simply balancing the scales.

It has been said that Kubler Ross' five stages of grief: denial, anger, bargaining, depression and acceptance extend to all forms of misfortune. While I was firmly stalled on the anger stage, George had landed in the acceptance stage in record time, and he worked tirelessly to get Noel set-up with the best professionals he could. Although I take some credit for Noel's diagnosis, George was the engine behind helping him. Five weeks after diagnosis, Noel had a speech therapist, an occupational therapist, a developmental pediatrician, and a developmental school.

Doors

"The door to success is opening. You will meet important people who will help you improve."

–Gillian Kemp & Mary Kuper
(What "doors" symbolize in tea leaves,
from *Tea Leaves, Herbs and Flowers.*)

"Health is infinite and expansive in mode, and reaches out to be filled with the fullness of the world; whereas disease is finite and reductive in mode, and endeavors to reduce the world itself."

–Oliver Sacks

Our world was suddenly under siege by what I like to call "the special needs police." The beautifully renovated Cape Cod-style home that was the source of so much tranquility and happiness a month prior was now overrun with therapists. Monday to Friday, they tracked through our home; many touting ideas of how the house should look, so as to create less external commotion for Noel.

"You need to get rid of all these toys."

"There's too much clutter."

"Can you take some things off the walls?" was their condemning chorus.

At the same time as giving instructions on home décor, alternatively, they always had a long list of things I was required to buy. The flux of outgoing toys vs. incoming toys seemed virtually the same, but I said nothing. As badly as I felt, I aimed to please, still believing that my willingness to go along with a professional's agenda was the key to Noel's success, a.k.a, my happiness.

For someone who was uncomfortable sharing space with a housekeeper once a week, adjusting to daily visits from therapists was torture. Their moods, my moods and Noel's progress, or rather, lack thereof, shaped each visit. Gone were the days when I could idly enjoy reading a book in the garden or put on some music at three in the afternoon and tango the kids from one side of the house to the other. My dream house had turned into a hospital waiting room, where I waited outside locked doors to hear the visiting therapist's report on my son. Occasionally, if I were out and arrived home to him working behind closed doors, I'd hear him ask for me. "Not until your work's done," the therapist's muffled voice behind the door would insist.

Home visits were pleasant in comparison to my new role as taxi driver. At one point, Noel had appointments in Woodland Hills (1x/week), Encino (2x/week), Culver City (4x/week), Westwood (3x/week), and Santa Monica (4x/week). Not only did this mean the bulk of time I spent alone with Noel was on the freeway, but it also meant that we were often away from Julian. Although Julian was much happier playing with friends at the playground, as opposed to sleeping the hours away on long freeway trips (he was at an age when he napped whenever fastened into a car seat), in retrospect, this may have contributed to his feeling insecure, always seeing Mom leaving with his brother, him being left out.

For a child with developmental delays, a standard pediatrician does not suffice. Your child needs a developmental pediatrician too. So, you make some calls and get an appointment. Easy. Except that the appointment isn't until nearly a year later. Like every profession that services people with autism, the medical field is severely understaffed. California has one of the highest incidences of autism (Pesce, Poindexter, Smith, and Zarembo), and in Los Angeles there are only a handful of developmental pediatricians to treat them. Consequently, they all have waiting lists.

But there are shortcuts. Having a tenacious husband is one of them. Here again, George was relentless in his pursuit of getting an appointment and within three months, we got Noel in to see Dr. R., another long car ride away, in La Canatta. A developmental pediatrician is the equivalent of a general contractor; they oversee the whole operation, which in this case is all your kid's services, including, prescribing multiple medications regardless of a child's age. Dr. R. had a doctor in Chicago with whom she worked closely, neurologist Dr. M. Even though he too was overbooked with appointments, she got us in to see him quickly.

All this expediency felt promising.

We packed our bags and headed to Chicago. Dr. M. believed there was a connection between seizures and autism, and he administered an overnight EEG to Noel. My career as "professional distracter" was born. While the nurse applied the glue to cover Noel's head with electrodes, I distracted him with cute phrases from his favorite Teletubby video, and a rousing chorus of "I've been working on the Railroad," complete with Noel's favorite bit, when I hold the "Fiddly-I-OOOOOOOOO!" We covered his head with a hat and kept him within range of the box recording his brain waves for 24-hours by sticking within the confines of our antiseptic rental apartment in a wealthy suburb of Chicago. George and I slept with Noel and the box in between us, if sleep is the word one uses to call closing one's eyes, but never quite losing consciousness.

The next day, Dr. M. said, "No other doctor would see seizures, but I do." He prescribed Depakote, an anti-seizure medication in conjunction with Prednisone, a steroid. When his or her child is ill, a parent will do virtually anything to help. Although I was more inclined to Eastern medicine, we'd had a friend of a friend talk to us for over an hour one evening, extolling the virtues of what Dr. M's work had done for his son.

"Let me be very clear," he said in an authoritative voice. "Dr. M. cured my son. The autism is gone. That word does not apply to my son anymore."

The past three months had been a litany of firsts for me. Why not add another? Although going against my core beliefs and putting Noel on medication was not easy, I did it. But as willing as I was to give the Depakote a try, I wouldn't agree to the steroid.

Like Sleeping Beauty, Noel slept most of the year he was on Depakote. In retrospect, he was barely alive, napping whenever possible and spending his waking hours in a perpetual state of lethargy. George was pre-med in college and put a lot of faith in Western medicine. I knew George would have some long, drawn-out method for stopping Depakote. I, on the other hand, hated every single day I added it to Noel's juice. Feeling like Mia Farrow in *Rosemary's Baby*, I had one goal in mind, to protect my child.

Without George knowing, I slowly stopped the Depakote to gauge Noel's reaction.

"Like a new child."

"He was over-medicated."

"The best he's ever been," his teachers and therapists said.

Armed with Noel's dramatic improvement post-Depakote, I finally told George. Although he couldn't argue with the positive results, he continues to remind me of my trickery to this day. Dr. M.'s reaction?

"It would have worked if you'd used the Prednisone" and "I have this new drug I'd like you to try..." Noel probably lost a year of development on Depakote, something he could scarcely afford.

An Individualized Education Plan (IEP), or what George and I have come to know as "the worst day of the year," is required by law for every child with special needs. Parents, teachers, therapists and school district personnel meet in the child's classroom. Surrounded by pictures of your child sitting alongside his classmates (any interaction with another child will suffice), and seeing his name on various pieces of primary colored artwork push-pinned to the walls, parents are lulled into a state of hope for normalcy. Then the meeting starts. For close to three hours, you have the surreal experience of sitting and listening to a cast of upwards of fifteen professionals—many whom you've never met—tell you everything your child *can't* do. The worst of it is, the school district (led by a particularly unsavory, maudlin older woman named Rose, in our case) tries to conserve its resources and denies parents as many services as possible.

We were lucky. After fighting the district on every point, George and our advocate were victorious. Noel got everything we asked for. Sadly, even our successes could be construed as disheartening. I couldn't help feeling Noel's poor performance was ultimately what got us the extra services.

Walls

Some ancient cultures do not step on ants or destroy a colony of them, because they believe a nest close to home is a sign of future wealth.

Europeans think Americans are obsessed with happiness. In *Something for Nothing*, Jackson Lears says, "A providential sense of destiny could be expanded from individuals to groups and ultimately to nations—and to none more easily than the United States. Prosperity itself came to seem a sign of God's blessing" (3).

A lifetime of good fortune had ill-prepared me for the challenges of hard luck. My internal mantra had changed from *Someone has to win, why not me?* to *Why did this have to happen to me?* Sadness was only outdone by a profound sense of self-pity.

I became careless.

The year after Noel was diagnosed, I had three car accidents, lost my wallet twice, and left things everywhere. I stopped wearing a seatbelt. Got sick every six weeks. The cats went from pampered bliss to barely being fed. I even got some satisfaction from drowning with Ajax the perennial parade of ants that made its way into our home sometime around Labor Day. For a lifelong vegetarian who routinely picked up strays and removed bugs found in the house to a safe spot outdoors, this was an extreme shift. Blanca, our El Salvadorian nanny, spoke very poor English, so I stopped talking to her. It was too much effort. On weekends, when Blanca wasn't there to tend to household chores, it was difficult to tell we had hardwood floors, since virtually every square foot was littered with toys, clothes and miscellaneous household debris.

I withdrew.

One of my accidents took place on Mother's Day, which I can only assume was directly related to my dismay that the day went largely ignored by George. I thought perhaps he too had become careless, until he eventually wished me a lackluster "Happy Mother's Day." Having my husband barely acknowledge me on Mother's Day wasn't the real problem. I felt invisible to him. Or rather, more like his assistant. His frequent phone calls to check on how Noel was doing, his demands to know specifics of every report, at the same time he was un-willing to hear bad news.

"He didn't too well," I would say.

"But he did okay, right?" He'd insist.

Worse was his utter resentment of any time I took for myself. "You don't have your writing class tonight, do you?" He'd say every week.

My answer was always the same. "Yes, I have it today as I have every Tuesday for the last two years."

When he questioned me on anything, I sulked, believing, because I was in crisis mode, I was beyond reproach.

I put up walls.

While it's true that all parents give up part of their lives for their children, when you have a child that is autistic, you give up your dreams too. Wondering if your child will be a good student, maybe an athlete or an artist, whether he'll marry and give you grandkids, becomes meaningless. Now, the only goal is for him to be "normal."

The repetitive hand motion that had been the alarm clock for his autism is called perseverating, or "stimming" and most kids with autism do it in one form or another. In *The Child with Special Needs*, writers Stanley Greenspan, M.D. and Serena Wieder, P.h.D. say, "This behavior is often an attempt to compensate for sensory underactivity, to seek extra sensation in order to register input" (150). Some stim with their eyes, intensely tracking an object up and down; many flap their hands, and oftentimes, stimming is accompanied by some bizarre vocalization, for the more severe, it can be a yell; some stims incorporate eyes, hands and voice (Greeenspan and Wieder 150).

As difficult as it was to diagnose Noel, a year after his diagnosis, there was no mistaking him for a typical child. He didn't play with other children, he spoke in one-word sentences, he had a chronic sinus infection that caused green snot to spew from his nose every eight weeks or so, he barely ate, never interacted with his brother Julian, and stimmed for long periods of the day.

In an age when it's hard to differentiate between schizophrenics, actors rehearsing lines, and cell phone users on the street, you'd think society would be willing to turn a blind eye to a small child with a nervous tic. But as Nathaniel Hawthorne said, "Men of cold passions have quick eyes" (Douglas). As much as I know that it's human nature, friends acted oddly around Noel. Clusters of parents speaking in lowered voices to one another were the norm whenever we were at social engagements. A blaring announcement on a megaphone couldn't have made the topic of their discussion more obvious. Even when a friend was exceptionally nice to Noel, I'd end up feeling bad. They'd asked Noel twenty ques-tions, not knowing that answering questions is the biggest hurdle of all for someone with autism. Like enemies outside a stone fortress wall, words seem impenetrable to the autistic brain. If he happened to answer a few questions, they'd praise his progress. If he didn't answer at all, they'd say nothing. While the praise felt patronizing, the lack of it was worse.

As Julian got older, the differences between him and Noel became more pronounced. Not only did we have one child that was typical and another neurotypical, in almost every aspect of their personalities, they were different. Julian liked play, Noel was incapable of it. Julian talked non-stop, Noel spoke very little. Julian loved interacting with his friends, Noel only interacted with adults. Being alone with the two of them was a challenge, since they both had very different ideas of how they wanted to spend their time. I often felt like I had twins in the physical sense: having to carry them both, changing diapers (Noel still wasn't potty trained), dressing and doing everything one does for toddlers. But the bond that twins share, or even brothers, was missing from their relationship. In the playground, I'd sprint back and forth from the monkey bars, where Julian was, to the outskirts of the playground, where Noel was fixated on the wheels of the assorted baby strollers. On the rare occasion when they agreed to the same activity—like going on the swings—inevitably, I'd encounter some other obstacle, like not being able to get two swings in a row. The other mothers somehow missed the desperate, maniacal look on my face. Many times, I failed to bridge the divide between their worlds.

It took me a while to realize that whenever I was having a really bad day, it was always related to how Noel was doing. The slightest negative report would leave me in a funk. The hardest times were those when he would do poorly for weeks at a time. Keeping up appearances was about the only thing I had energy for. The reality of our lives was much different than the facade. Some days, my heart felt so heavy, the extra weight made it hard to lift my feet.

I turned to my no-fail system of coping with a problem: acquiring knowledge through reading. Therapists or doctors would recommend that I read this article or that book, saying, "This person is amazing! You'll feel better after you read this." I dutifully would track down said book or article, expecting to feel consoled, inspired, hopeful. Wrong. The more I read about people with autism, the more depressed I became. I took little comfort in reading that Temple Grandin comforted herself with a self-invented squeeze machine, or that autistic persons had to relearn driving every time they got behind the wheel—most people with autism don't drive.

In *The Child with Special Needs,* autistic persons are described in this way:

> Some children with autistic spectrum disorders are also labeled mentally retarded because many of the component skills are severely affected. Other children are considered autistic but have unusual abilities. They may be able to memorize whole books or carry out certain mathematical operations, they may even be precocious in some areas, such as reading—but they can't connect intent or emotion to these component parts and thus give purpose and meaning to the way they function. (Greenspan and Wieder 342)

For the first time in my life, reading failed me.

Bad luck has a way of following bad. The worst day post-diagnosis occurred on a sunny Thursday morning, when George and I had an appointment with Noel's occupational therapist, Ms. G. Of all the professionals who worked with Noel, we trusted her opinion the most. We expected she was going to discuss his good progress, since he'd had positive reports of late, or maybe a conversation about kindergarten, just four months away. George always begins appointments with small banter, a sign of what a true optimist he is. I, on the other hand, sit tensed, feeling the shoes on my feet, and with my hands, the surface of the table in front of me. Mindful of the bad news she's about to deliver, thankfully, Ms. G. doesn't let George go on forever. She interrupts him, leans forward looking from George to me and says, "I have to tell you, I think there's some M.R."

Roof

> "70% of children with autism have some mental retardation."
> —Michael D. Powers

The sad truth about diagnosing a child with a developmental delay is that immediately, you see them differently. They're no longer your beautiful baby who delights you with the slightest action or expression. A lot of the time, the label is all you see.

When Noel was diagnosed with autism, I had to fall in love with him again. When Ms. G. labeled him as having some mental retardation, I had to do it *all over again.*

Falling in love isn't easy for those whose emotions have been deadened. One way to learn to love again is through the eyes of others. Admittedly, this is corny stuff. But when you are in crisis, it's surprising how useful clichés become.

I have never met another father more in love and more involved with his children than George. Through all our trials and tribulations, he has worked tirelessly to help Noel. Other fathers of children with special needs do a fraction of what he does, if they stick around at all. I wish I could accurately describe the way George's eyes light up when Noel walks into the room, but you'll just have to trust me. And then there's Julian. For all their differences, Julian is Noel's fiercest protector. When we were in New York waiting for the subways, Julian stood by Noel, to make sure he stayed clear of the tracks and got off and on the train in time. When he's around new friends, Julian puts his arm around Noel and says with great pride, "He's my brother!" And Noel's relationship with my mother is something very special. Sometimes when I'm having a hard day, I think of my mother's love for Noel and feel better. He is, simply put, the light of her life.

Luckily, Ms. G's diagnosis was proved wrong. And Noel isn't hard to love. Through the years, the roof of our expectations for Noel has slowly been raised. Occasionally, we get a glimpse of the sky. Turns out, he really is answering all the questions asked him, just inside his head.

There's a poetry to Noel's autism: the way he sees mathematical patterns in his head; memorizes the birthday of every person he's ever met; has learned to read by reading street signs and bus schedules; his undeniable need to touch someone when he sleeps; the enthusiastic way he greets people he knows; his love for babies and sleeping people; his intense love of being immersed in any body of water (be it bath or ocean); his adorable little face, framed with a haircut Paul McCartney would envy and cheeks sun-kissed with freckles; his adventurous spirit for travel and trying new things; his unrestrained belly laugh at slapstick; the little hop dances he does that makes his bangs bob up and down; the way he pretends he knows the words to songs and sing/hums along regardless; and most of all, his boundless love for family.

Sure, I'm worried about the day when Noel hits adolescence. Behaviors that were cute and different in a baby somehow become weird and menacing in an adolescent. Hopefully, love will see us through, as it has thus far.

Some say children with special needs are closer to God. Others say the misfortune we have in this life is retribution from the last. While I would never say I feel lucky to have a child with special needs, I will say—as many who've met Noel have echoed—if there is such a thing as angels among us, Noel is certainly one of them. And that must be lucky.

Resources

Eisenberg, Arlene and Heidi Murkoff. *What to Expect: The Toddler Years.* New York: Workman Publishing, 1994. Print.

Greenspan, Stanley, I., and Serena Wieder. *The Child With Special Needs: Encouraging Intellectual and Emotional Growth.* Jackson, TN: Perseus Books, 1998. Print.

Douglas, Charles Noel. "Forty Thousand Quotations: Prose and Poetical." *Bartleby.com.* Bartleby.com, 2012. Web. 15 Aug. 2013.

Lears, Jackson. *Something for Nothing.* New York, NY: Penguin, 1947. Print.

Pesce, Anthony, Sandra Poindexter, Doug Smith, and Alan Zarembo. "Autism Rates by State." *Los Angeles Times.* Los Angeles Times, 9 Dec. 2011. Web. 15 Aug. 2013.

ParentPals.com. Parentpals.com, 2012. Web. 15 Aug. 2013.

Powers, Dr. Michael. *Children with Autism: A Parents Guide.* Bethesda, MD: Woodbine House, 1989. Print.

Grandin, Temple. *Thinking in Pictures: and Other Reports from My Life with Autism.* New York, NY. First Vintage Books Edition, 1996. Print.

Fragments of the First Five Days

Jane Dwyer

Day 1

Sage is airlifted from the ER to Children's Hospital, three hours after his home birth. When the flight crew takes him from my arms, I ask for pain medication. Something, anything to quiet the screaming muscles of my body so I can follow him to Seattle. They comply. I am placed in a darkened room to rest and the soothing touch of an angelic nurse calms me. Later, they attempt to repair my shredded perineum.

I lose the rest of the day.

A photo proves I made the journey back to him.

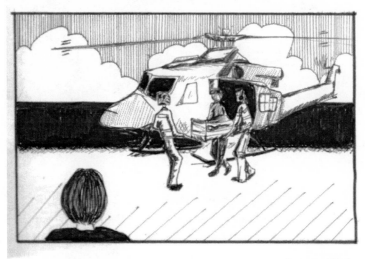

Bridgette Shively

Day 2

Neonatal intensive care. Sage in an isolette. The heels of his tender feet purple from the needle sticks for blood samples. Looking down at Sage, the craniofacial Doctor is explaining the future to me. Sage's body stiffens, he arches his back, he stops breathing...he starts again. A seizure? A flurry of activity, a spinal tap. "Do you want to hold your baby during the procedure?" "No." IV antibiotics are started. When they are finished, I hold him. I do not put him down.

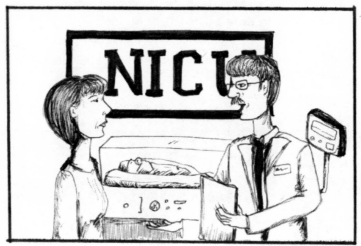

Bridgette Shively

Day 3

I spend the nights on a hard torture rack of a futon at my friend's house. My body is one huge throbbing pulse. Sage's kidneys have shut down. A thread of a catheter is inserted through his tiny penis into his bladder to monitor his urine output. I am beaten. I wander out of the NICU and sit on the flat green bench in front of the elevators. The pinging of the doors opening and closing lulls me over and down into sleep. I dream that Sage's diaper is wet. He has peed around his catheter. I am nursing him and when I look down he is a monkey, milk spilling down his chin. I know he is brain damaged. I am horrified. I wake up, my face stuck to the plastic cushion. I lock the monkey image far away.

I return to the unit, to find his catheter has been removed. "He wet his diaper, urinated around the tube," the excited nurse tells me.

I gather him in my arms. I rock him the rest of the day.

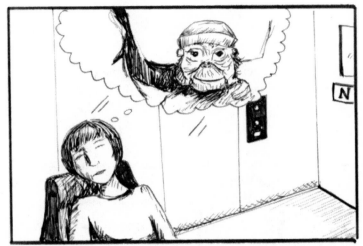

Bridgette Shively

Day 4

Sage is discharged to pediatrics. The anticonvulsant medication has made him too sleepy to feed regularly. A tube is passed through his mouth into his stomach and formula administered with a syringe. His input and output are carefully measured. He is taken for a CAT scan and when he returns his body temperature is subnormal. An incubator is ordered. "No," I say, "no more." I tuck him down onto my bare chest, wrap us in warm blankets. His temperature returns to normal.

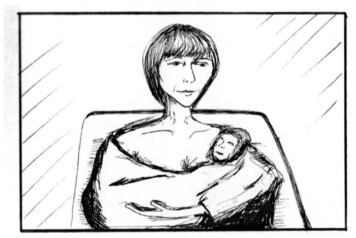

Bridgette Shively

Day 5

    To be released, I must demonstrate that I can tube feed Sage. I shut off my emotions, and complete the procedure flawlessly. When asked about his bottle intake and how many wet diapers he's produced, I tell them the amount they want to hear. We are discharged.

    Posed in front of a sign announcing where we have been, a photo shows Sage held tightly in my arms, my face lit up, my smile real.

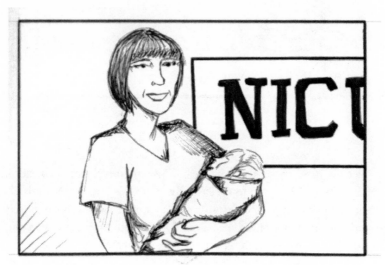

Bridgette Shively

Stopped Holding My Breath

Carmen Iwaszczenko

And what does a parent of a child like ours have to forgive? A lot. Many times over. Years and years of "well-meaning" comments from family members, friends, coworkers, teachers, people at doctors' and dentists' offices, and people in check-out lines—eventually become a pile of concern and anxiety. He talked too loudly, he chewed sloppily, he bounced and rocked, he was clumsy, he didn't pick up after himself, he talked too much sometimes, he didn't talk enough, he didn't say "hello" when someone said it to him, he got easily distracted, he shied away from kids too much, he was in other kids' personal space too much, he broke things, he was too curious, he was excitable, he touched things he shouldn't, he fought too much with his sister, he had to be told too many times; he was a "handful."

He was my son.

Rudeness, annoyance, and very little understanding were often encountered. I have been told that children who don't look disabled on the outside often have these sorts of misunderstandings. Another time we had an older woman on a transfer bus between Disney parks in Florida make a comment on how little he spoke back to her when she was trying to chat up some small talk with him.

"He must be worn out," she said.

I told her he has autism. She clammed up nearly instantly, and then tried to recover by sharing how well he was doing in light of that information. This from a woman who buzzed to the front of an extensive boarding line with her motorized scooter and took up about one eighth of the bus by parking her scooter and sitting in a bus seat beside it. Her handicap apparently was allowance for her to bypass others like ourselves—and we were the very last people to be able to fit aboard that particular bus. One bus seat was left, so I placed my son there (next to scooter woman), because his balance isn't the best and standing during a bus ride would be precarious for him. My husband, myself, and my four-year-old daughter would stand. We thought this was better than waiting another twenty minutes for another bus. It probably was, because the next bus might have held yet another misunderstanding anyways.

The cut that hurt the most came that first Christmas after the diagnosis. It still remains the pinnacle of disgust in my history of "family" behavior.

My mother had cancelled our Christmas celebration that year, saying that she felt she couldn't celebrate without my dad who died the same year we were dealing with our son's new diagnosis (label). It broke her children's hearts—but we celebrated separately, even though the custom was to all be packed together under our parents' roof. All of us siblings called each other that day to say how crazy this was—to be skipping Christmas—and how awful it felt; and we also said how we wouldn't let it be like that again next year.

The flip side of this coin was something most married couples know well enough—the in-laws' celebration. Knowing that we weren't required anywhere else that year, my mother-in-law had called us over early to help her cook and get ready for the whole family. We lived the closest and went over to oblige her request. We also hadn't learned to say no yet.

Dinner for the family was scheduled for 4:00 pm. We were there at 2:00 pm. Our two kids were very excited and were told they couldn't touch anything in the mountain of presents under the tree until they finished their dinner—which was hours away. They were ages seven and three at the time and having a hard time waiting while mommy and daddy were busy helping cook and get ready for a big Christmas dinner. My mother-in-law had also asked if I would take a family portrait, so I was setting up my camera and tripod in the basement.

As dinnertime approached, the other family members started to arrive. And then 4:00 pm would come and go with my husband's youngest sister calling to say she'd be late. Twenty minutes later she came, and most of us had started supper without her family. In our case, the children had been waiting for hours to get supper over with to get to those presents! So they were squirrely and excited and rushed through dinner and started to move around the house in anticipation. And my husband and I did very little to "correct" them, because they were young, and they had been patient enough in our eyes—and we saw little to correct. Yet, that youngest sister of my husband—she couldn't sit back and relax (though she rarely can, anyway). She felt the need to correct every little misstep (especially of my son) that evening. But she wasn't even trying to be nice about it. Maybe it was because she had an eight-month old of her own, or because she and her husband were not getting along, or maybe it's just because she's a perfectionist type A-1 bitch with little else to do but bully her own brother's children—whatever the reason, she felt the need to ride my son's ass that evening.

She nervously walked around with her fake "oh so sweet" voice saying the meanest things. Things like, "if these were my kids, I'd remove sugar from their diets completely." After a half a dozen like comments and a bunch of her movement towards trying to get our kids to "settle down" by moving them to a different table to try to get them to color some coloring pages, my husband finally got up and lost his temper. There was all out verbal warfare launched between the two of them with the whole family around. My husband would tell her that our kid needed to practice social skills and she would reply that a family gathering was no place to do that (which made my blood boil, by the way).

"And I suppose *your* kids are perfect?!" my husband would say indignantly, and much too loudly for a Christmas supper. To which she would reply, "Yes they *are*" (No shit, I could barely believe it myself). And he would rebut, "I suppose that's why your [12-year-old] daughter mouths off so much to her grandparents? That's *perfect* behavior!"

Of course, the argument was going way south of "constructive" by this point, and I was promptly told to go get my coat and get the kids dressed in theirs—we were leaving.

So I did—I went for coats and dressed them up and the whole while there was a bunch of back and forth between bully and her brother—and now some other interjections to calm down from other family members. My husband's voice was booming upstairs as I went downstairs and collected my photography equipment. Coming back up, cuss words were now being interjected, and children were now crying, but no one, not a one of them, not even my husband's parents—none of them did anything to stand up for us. They let the youngest daughter play bully to us on Christmas. I was the last one heading for the door, and I said to my husband's parents that I was sorry, and that I really didn't know what to do. My husband was out in the van already with the kids waiting for me. I tried to tell my sister-in-law that our son would need more understanding in coming years, and that if she couldn't cope, then our family would not be able to attend family gatherings anymore.

And the last thing I would do is try to leave a thought in his sister's head about what kind of understanding we need. I said to her, "our son has a disability."

She replied, "that's NO EXCUSE!"

And with that, I shook my head in tears and disbelief and I walked out the door, closing it behind me. I felt so betrayed. What's worse is how my husband and son felt.

We'd go home with two kids in tears with wide-open mouths lamenting about not being able to open presents before we left. And when we got home, my husband went out in the winter cold for a half an hour walk to collect himself while I dealt with the kids' disappointment.

My daughter would cry to me, "why can't we open presents?"

And my son would respond to her, "because daddy and his sister were fighting!"

And I asked my son if he knew why they were fighting. He said, "half because of me, and half because they are crazy."

I thought to myself, "wow." He took my breath away with the accuracy of that response.

In so few words he'd told me that first off, he knows that his existence was related to this bad thing had happening. And secondly, he knew well enough that what he'd seen was indeed crazy behavior for a family! Anger *burned* in me. "I can't let *anyone* let my kid think that they are the cause of *bullshit* like that," I thought. "I miss my dad," another inner cry slipped into my head. I wished very much at that moment that I could pick up the phone and talk to Dad. He always knew the right thing to say. He would have been the support I needed. But he was no more. My husband and I would lie together and cry before going to sleep that night.

A day later I would tell my mother-in-law that we wouldn't stand for anyone treating us (especially our son) that way, and that I expected an apology from her daughter; I was disappointed and felt betrayed that she or her husband hadn't stood up for us and helped stop the argument that night, especially since it was under their roof. She didn't have much to say, except for her daughter shouldn't have said those things, her daughter was under so much stress, and that she'd talk to her. We haven't had a similar instance, though we barely make time to interact with the bully sibling anymore. The relationship between her and my husband was scarred forever that night.

I also told my mother-in-law that if she needed help in the future preparing, that she would have to call upon someone else. I told her that for us, it is very difficult to be there for that long and have the kids under expectation to behave perfectly for the entire duration. In essence, I was saying "no" to any future requests before they were even made. It was a difficult line to draw, but it's an appropriate boundary to set. All things considered, it was necessary and the right thing to do. It took the anger and betrayal to give me the guts to say "no" to her this way. I wish we'd had the sense to say no before that. Things may have turned out so differently. It wasn't a selfish thing, really, to say "no" to her. In our circumstance, it was a necessary thing. Yet we feared upsetting my mother-in-law, or disappointing her, or leaving her be overwhelmed in a situation she wasn't ready to handle on her own.

I like to call this the Insanity Summit Christmas of 2011. Not to be confused with the Insanity Summit of 2008 (another entirely outlandish story of dysfunction). So yes, there was a history of ridiculousness—and a disabled child coming into that picture is truly a recipe for disaster. The passage of time has mended the relationships to some extent, but a hell of a lot of trust went by the wayside in these events.

In telling our psychologist about these encounters, I was advised to only "hang out" with people who have less pathology than we do. In other words, we didn't have enough of time or extra emotional strength to deal with other people's problems. She said that people like us, with the challenges we had lying before us, needed to learn to surround ourselves with helpful, supportive people. We couldn't be spending our time on someone else's problems, because we would be very busy just figuring out our own day-to-day solutions. It's been some of the best advice I've received related to our situation to date.

I have yet to hear any inkling of an apology about the Insanity Summit Christmas, first-hand or otherwise. I've decided not to hold my breath. But in the end, the most important lesson that we've learned through that experience was that we cannot let our son's disability be mistaken for misbehavior. Like any other parents, we have to be his constant advocates and protectors—but perhaps to a higher degree. I know there will be many opportunities to experience the stigma related to my son's autism. I wish there was a way to save our son and ourselves from the hurt that will come along with those instances. I know I cannot take each one to heart, or I'll be eaten up alive by anger and resentment. I have to be able to forgive, to move on, to choose my battles better, and to live the best life we can together.

Opening Doors
Robin LaVoie

I am standing on my back patio, watching my five-year-old son through the sliding glass door. He is bouncing around the kitchen on his large blue exercise ball, happily unaware that he has just locked his mother out of the house.

He didn't mean to lock me out. I had stepped outside—just for a moment—to throw something away, and I left the door open. After I went around the corner of the house, Blake simply returned the door to its "normal" state: closed, with the latch pointed down. That's how the door always looks when he is inside. Like many other autistic people, my child is very aware of his surroundings and tends to "fix" things that are out of place. Lights on that should be off, books rearranged on shelves, doors left open that must be closed, and latches returned to their down and locked positions.

"Unlock the door, Blake," I say, shaking the door handle. He rolls his ball over to the door and presses his palms against the glass. He grins at me and sits back down on his ball. I instruct him: "Pull *up*," and mime lifting the latch. He slides off the ball and copies my hand motions. But he doesn't touch the handle.

"OPEN DOOR, Blake," I demand, failing in my attempt to keep the growing worry out of my voice. My son laughs and repeats, "Open door, Blake!" But he doesn't understand.

It all comes down to this—all the hours of behavioral and speech therapy, doctors' appointments, IEP meetings and filing cabinets full of data sheets and treatment goals. If my son cannot understand a simple instruction to unlock the door, what does it matter if he knows his colors, his shapes? If he can recite the alphabet forwards and backwards? What does it matter if he expands his limited verbal ability to place "I want" before a request for juice or a cookie, if he cannot comprehend my words when he is in danger?

I run across the street to my neighbor's house to call my sister-in-law, who is the only person with a spare key, since my husband is out of town. She doesn't answer. I race back home, convinced that Blake will either be crying since I am missing or, what is more likely, getting himself into some kind of trouble. I find him perfectly content in the air-conditioned house, bouncing on his ball near the kitchen table, taking bites of his lunch. *Dear God, please don't choke.*

I go back to my neighbor's house to call a locksmith, cursing myself for not hiding a key outside. The locksmith says he can be here in twenty minutes. How many things can go wrong in twenty minutes?

I return to my patio, to wait where I can play with Blake through the glass and try every so often to get him to let me in. The hazards of my once child-safe kitchen are clear from my new vantage point. I begin to strategize. Which window can I break if he grabs that sharp knife off the counter or if he climbs up on the still warm stove? Can I throw this metal patio chair hard enough to break the glass if he falls off that damned ball and cracks his head on the hard tile floor? Oblivious to the threats that surround him, Blake laughs and bounces and taps on the glass between us.

Just as I reassure myself that at least I can keep an eye on him, my kid leaves the room. He runs into my bedroom where, of course, the window blinds are closed. I cannot see him, but I can hear him jumping on the bed, a favorite pastime that I instantly redefine as reckless. I hear him yell "Jumponthebed!"—one of the rare times he calls for me to play. I am helpless to respond.

Then, it happens. My son reappears, running into the kitchen and over to me at the door. He pulls on the handle, notices the latch and—without hesitation—flips it up and slides the door open. I am stunned by the speed at which my dilemma is solved. Blake, in turn, is bewildered by his mother's enthusiastic and borderline hysterical response. I cry and hug and sigh, and he just smiles, as if to say, *It's about time, Mom, what were you doing outside for so long?*

It is not always about ability. More often it is about motivation. My child could easily learn how to unlock the door; he just needed a *reason.* People with autism spectrum disorders often have difficulty seeing the world from another's perspective—*my* need to get inside did not register with Blake. Until it became *his* need, the locked door didn't concern him.

Years later, my interactions with my son are still shaped by this experience—besides, of course, moving the goal of teaching the meaning of "unlock" to the top of the priority list (and yes, hiding a spare key). The *most* important thing I can do is give my son ample reason to use and strengthen his abilities—and to discover what will entice and motivate him to open the doors that stand between us, waiting to be unlocked.

Risk Assessment

Kimberly Escamilla

Her phone voice can't mask the news.
Before the volta, before the pregnant pause

she unfurls a list of negatives—which are positives.
Sickle-cell, Tay-Sachs, Fragile x., Rh, Downs.

However,
Your placenta isn't producing protein. Low PAPP-A.

How can I take all those P's seriously.
But serious, she is.

My womb is a slum: leaky roof, bad plumbing.
Eggs at my age aren't prime real estate, I know.

This could be a sign of Trisomy 18,

Tri—there's a tercet, a third wheel, a hanger-on.
Later, Google terror sets in—*most end in miscarriage,*
extra fingers, no nose, heart on the wrong side.

Or not.

Instruction Manual
Sally Bittner Bonn

"You might consider taking Oscar to an orthopaedic specialist to have his spine checked. His kyphosis is getting worse. He might need a body jacket. At least to wear in his stander." Oscar's physical therapist is at the house for her weekly session.

I'm on the floor, back against the couch, begging it to hold me up. I say nothing.

Oscar lays on his side on the living room rug. Minnie, his PT, kneels over him, one hand flat against his spine, the other on his sternum, gently but firmly pressing her hands in and out toward one another. She is checking the flexibility of his spine. It's true, in an upright position he is hunching forward more and more. I'm sure she's right. I'm sure a body jacket would help him. But I can't do it. I can't take one more intervention, one more sign that my son's body is failing him. Actively. Aggressively. Isn't this supposed to happen later? Isn't it enough that I'm failing him?

With his arms outstretched, he plays with the rubber alligator she has brought him today, unaffected by our conversation.

"His spine is very supple. He has full movement. You can do this," indicating the movement of her hands, "to help his spine remain fluid." Her voice is upbeat, trying to soften the weight she dropped on me moments ago. She knows me well. My silence betrays me. Of course with all that's happened this week, anyone could read me like a grade school primer.

The room is open and filled with light from the large picture window. The blonde hardwood floors gleam all around the area rug. The six-foot by six-foot bookshelf is dwarfed in the large room. Yet the air is closing in around me. From above, from all sides. It's pressing in toward me and getting heavier and heavier. I'm trying to hold onto myself long enough to get through the PT session. My chest is so compressed, I can hardly get air in.

That's it. I'm failing him. He needs a body jacket because I haven't been doing trunk extension with him, I tell myself (never mind the natural progression of the disease). I'm also failing him because I don't know what to say when he says, "I wish I could walk like those guys," as two of his classmates walk past his wheelchair in the parking lot on the way into preschool. Or when he cries because he can't position his body the way he wants it. Like last week at nap.

I had settled him in, and he asked me to position Sully and Simon, his two stuffed animals, for snuggling. At age three he is excellent at giving directions, but no matter what I did, it just wasn't right. He was frustrated and started crying.

"I wish Sully could just move into position by himself and he didn't need to have people move him around." I understood immediately that he was talking about himself.

"You know, none of your other stuffed animals can move around by themselves, can they? Does it make you sad that sometimes another person has to move them into position?"

"Yes." More tears.

"Does that make you think of yourself?"

"Yes." A big flood of tears.

"It's okay to be sad."

He cries and cries. I lie down next to him and try to snuggle him.

"Sit up. Sit up," he manages to choke out between gulps of air. I sit up, and he keeps crying. I feel completely helpless. I sit still, my eyes darting around the room for an answer.

"Would you like me to hold you?"

"Yes."

Ah. Relief. This I can do. I scoop him up and ask if he'd like to rock in the rocking chair in mama and dada's room. He does. And we do. His lengthening three-year-old body draped down my adult mama body. We rock and rock and rock and soothe both our souls.

"Sing, Mama." I'm not the musical one in the family. I have exactly two songs in my repertoire: "Twinkle, Twinkle, Little Star" and "Somos El Barco," a dual-language folk song from my childhood. Oscar's not interested in either. He wants me to make up songs about light. And beads. And dinosaurs and characters. Steering into unchartered waters, I do. We laugh a little and calm down. Ease back toward nap. I settle him in his bed, and he goes to sleep. But I walk away at a loss. How on earth does a mother answer her son's cries that his body can't do what other people's bodies can do?

Surely there must be a book. A series of articles. Some sort of guide that gives parents of disabled children a tiny little hint of how to respond to your three year-old when he says these things. I began asking when Oscar was still two and wasn't yet really talking about his differences. We knew it was coming, though. As young as 26 months,

he said one night, around the Christmas tree, "Oscar stand up by self."
But no one I talked to seemed to have the answer I was looking for.

I started with Families of SMA, the incredibly supportive national organization for people affected by Oscar's disease. They had reached out to us upon his diagnosis with brochures and even a care package. They'd been willing to help on a number of levels, from advice for a family fundraiser to welcoming us with open arms when we met them face-to-face at the national conference for the first time. Surely they must have some material that helps parents know how to talk with their children about disability. They sent me a long list that included books on how to set up a special needs trust, how to manage medical care for a special needs child, transitioning to adulthood with a disability, as well as reflections from family members about living with a special needs child. I felt overwhelmed and didn't explore the list any further.

I asked our service coordinator, who was a social worker working for a state-wide agency that services children with special needs. Surely the agency must have resources available. She said she'd do some research and get back to me. She had to go digging. She came back, several weeks later, with an eleven-page list of children's books, mostly about autism and other issues that didn't relate in any way to our situation. She highlighted a few she thought might apply most to Oscar, but still had no ideas or resources for me about my part in responding to Oscar. What I'm supposed to say, or not say, to my child about disability. No insight on how to meet him where he is.

We mentioned this to Oscar's neurologist, this difficulty in finding information, guidance for parents. Surely a physician could point us in the right direction. She said there's no money in it. No one wants to fund the research because there's no money to be made. Drugs. There's money in developing drugs and treatments. But, but my mind is sputtering. These are incurable diseases! Don't people need to know how to live day-to-day?! How to have an emotionally healthy and enriching life while they wait for years and years for drugs, which may never come down the pipeline and may or may not improve their physical condition?

In desperation, after the naptime episode, I call the nurse practitioner who works with one of Oscar's doctors. She does community outreach, in-services in schools. She must know something. Here's an untapped resource, surely. She agrees to do some research and get back to me. Twenty-five minutes later the phone rings, and it's her! Wow! How quick! She gives me the title of two children's books.

Sigh. I look them up, and they look really good, and I vow to check them out of the library, but they are still not going to tell me what to say to my son when he is lying on the floor crying because he doesn't have the strength to hold himself up on his elbows like his parents do, like his friends do, like babies much smaller and less coordinated than he can.

I don't need a book that's going to open the door to a conversation. The door is already wide open. Oscar has done that much. Now what am I supposed to do? Just listen? Console him? Tell him I'm sorry? Am I supposed to redirect his energy toward what he can do? Distract him by telling him other kids are envious of his wheels? What? I'd be delighted, even, to read a book with solid advice I strongly disagree with. At least this would give me direction. Show me what I don't want to do. Any stories of how parents have approached this subject in the past. Any opinion would give me something to chew on. But there's nothing! No one has any advice for me. At this point, I've had it.

So, a week after the naptime episode, which has left me devastated, I find myself in the midst of this disastrous day, overwhelmed by jumbled thoughts and feelings. I've been crying. Sobbing. I feel like I'm failing my son. David and I, who always work so well together as a team, are fighting. Neither of us is sleeping because we each get out of bed five, seven, who-knows-how-many times because we've lost track, in the night, to roll Oscar over. I so desperately want a second child and can't imagine ever having the energy and all this has me a mess. And no one has any real ideas of how I should talk with my son, respond to his comments and tears. Now, this afternoon, our beloved PT who has become like family, is saying difficult things about my Oscar's spine.

"Minnie, it's been a hard week," my voice cracks and my eyes glass up. "He's starting to talk about what he can't do."

She settles. Centers. Looks right into my eyes. "And there will be tears."

"There already have been. I don't know what to do." There is a burning in my chest and throat. I'm trying so hard to hold the repaired floodgates in place.

"You have to cry with him, tell him it's not fair. He has to know that you understand his pain. You will never feel exactly what he feels, but you have to let him know you're sad, too. That you're there for him, with him."

The tension slowly slides from my shoulders, down my back and out of my body. My breath fills my chest more fully. The darkness crowding my temples backs off. The muscles in my throat release.

The answer is so simple. So real. I have been making desperate phone calls, sending emails, for months, yet no one could answer me. No doctor, no social worker, no nurse practitioner, no parent advocate. Only the wise PT who has special needs children of her own. I should have known she'd have the answer I need.

I am soaked in gratitude.

Show & Tell: Part I

Anna Yarrow

1.

"I love you"
is when my mom
sings bedtime songs
and tries to hug me
(but it hurts)
goodnight
turns off the light
and shuts the door.
But I never
say it back.

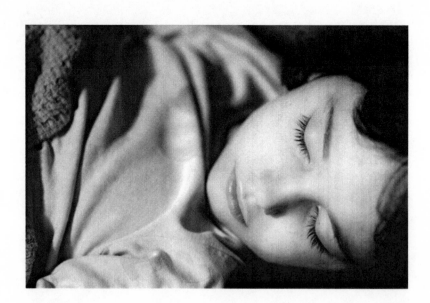

2.

"Why don't you go play?"
No.
I'll just
lay here and
remember my past
lives, which were
way better than
this.

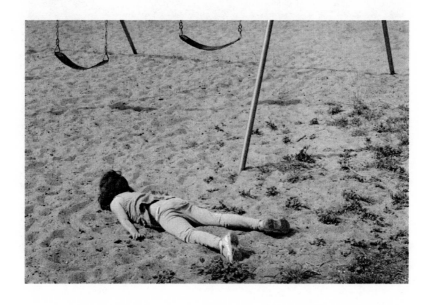

3.

She's not my real mom
because she makes me
clean my room
(I like it messy!)
and wear clothes to school
(I'd rather be naked!)
She doesn't *really* believe
I'm a T-rex
(dragon, dolphin, fairy, superhero)
from another planet
with special powers
to make her disappear.

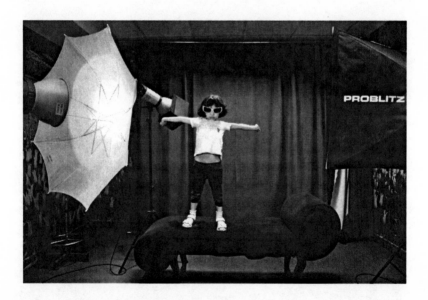

4.

I said I want to die
because it would
be peaceful
in a dark hole
and people would
stop bossing me.

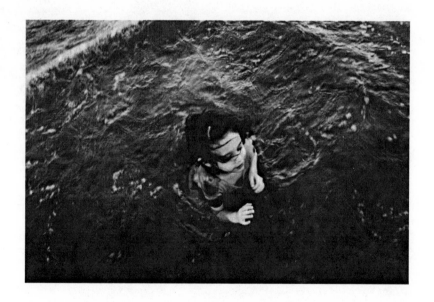

Happy Birthday
Christina K. Searcy

This is a picture of Daniel's third birthday. He looks so adorable blowing out the candles on his Dora the Explorer cake. He even looks like he has a smile on his face. There is Daddy, holding his big boy. This could be any preschool boy and any proud father. This is what you see in this picture.

What you don't see in this picture?

Immediately after this picture was taken and the candles were blown out, you can't hear the applause from his aunt, neighbors, and sisters. You can't see Daniel cry, "No clapping!" and start wailing. You can't see what happened ten minutes later, when the candles were removed, and we attempted to cut a slice out of the cake. It's hard to believe this adorable little boy became horror stricken from someone cutting his idol Dora's face. He wanted that piece returned to the cake plate immediately. In his mind, it belonged together and cutting it into pieces was repulsive and horrifying.

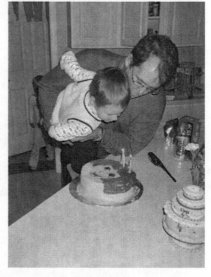

You don't see the frustration at being unable to verbalize his feelings, nor his confusion as to why his beloved Mommy and Daddy would so thoughtlessly consider defacing his long time hero. You cannot see his mad dash for the sliding glass door where the repetitive, consistent opening and closing would distract and calm him. The disappointment on Daniel's twin sister's face is absent from the picture, as she was learning at such a young age that her birthday was, mostly, not about her. Hidden from the picture are the hour of tears, spinning, and tantrums that followed and our desperate attempts to salvage a happy memory of the twins' third birthday.

I had not yet made peace with this life that was not picture-perfect. I had yet to admit that the family I expected was not my family and that not all memories need to be happy to be cherished. Looking back on this experience makes me now appreciate how far we have come—Daniel has grown, our family has foraged a new identity, and perhaps most of all, I have changed. The person I have become finds a cherished memory in what is real and not what was just pictured.

The Least of These: Caregiving in America
Barbara Crooker

Recently, I watched a segment on one of the morning news shows about a family with a child with a rare disease. The glossy anchorwoman was clucking sympathetically, as she said, "What makes this so difficult is that not only is there no cure, there is not even any treatment." And I thought, "Well, welcome to *my* world." I'm the mother of an adult son, age 28, with autism. Not only is there no cure and no treatment, but no one actually knows what autism IS, apart from a collection of symptoms. Autism isn't considered rare any more, as the rates have risen from one in 20,000 (rarer than most childhood cancers) to one in 125, so almost everyone knows someone, a neighbor, a relative, etc. with ASD (autism spectrum disorder). Yet every year, more and more children are diagnosed, while at the same time, states are cutting their budgets (special education is expensive), and there are few, if any, services available for adults with autism. We've gone, in our journey, from hearing that David is on a long waiting list for a group home to this: "*Maybe* I could get him a referral to a homeless shelter." This is what our previous social worker said, when I raised the "what if" (we both died tomorrow in a car crash) question. I hope you, dear reader, find this as shameful as I do, living as we do in a wealthy first world nation.

Our new social worker has tried to alleviate our concerns, saying that a group home is a more restrictive environment, and that what she'd recommend is something called "life sharing," which would mean placing David in a family home (rather like foster care, except he wouldn't be moved frequently, as he would if he were a child in the foster care system). My husband and I are "aging out"; he's 70 and I'm nearing 70, but how could we ever put our child, who we love dearly, in someone else's home? "Between a rock and a hard place you are," says Yoda.

But this is my life, and here are some of the gritty details. Our day begins at 5:30 am on David's sheltered workshop days, and at 4:45 am on the days he has his "community job" (code for "real" job, in shipping and receiving at a local department store). We have to provide transportation to and from work, as we live in a rural community, and there is no public transportation. So we, the parents, must do the driving, not only for work, but also for doctors, recreation, etc. We are "fortunate," in that his sheltered workshop is fully funded; younger clients now have to be funded by their own families to the tune of $7000 a year (in order to be piece workers, one step up from a sweatshop, albeit with nicer supervisors and working conditions). David's job usually consists of putting markers in a box, or blocks of clay in a carton (most of the work comes from Binney & Smith, the Crayola people), and he enjoys it, as he really likes repetition. In the department store, he unloads the truck, brings goods to various sections of the store, strips plastic off clothing, and recycles the boxes by crushing them. He hasn't been able to move beyond needing job coaching services (at the sheltered workshop, there is supervision on site), so we can't consider him a fully independent worker. The hope was that "natural supports" (code for "kind fellow employees") would take over the role of job coach, but that hasn't happened, at least not yet.

When he comes home, he is fairly independent. Earlier in the day, he has performed his "daily living" tasks, such as showering, dressing, preparing breakfast, making his lunch for work, by himself. We have had him on a gluten-free (no wheat, barley, oats, and rye) and casein-free (no dairy) diet, since he was eight years old, which means a great deal of planning, as many of his food items need to be special-ordered from websites, and most of his food is made from scratch. Often, I prepare two parallel, but separate, dinners (for example, rice spaghetti with meatballs made with gluten-free bread (and no cheese) for him, regular spaghetti and meatballs with Parmesan cheese for us), and I bake cookies for him weekly. This diet is key to his ability to function as well as he does (and was instrumental in his being able to complete his high school education), but is, as one might imagine, difficult to do. We have a cardinal rule, "if it's illegible (i.e., if there's no labeling), it's inedible," so that he doesn't have any "slips," and he is sometimes a better label reader than I am, as my eyes age.

We also have to constantly monitor his behavior, trying to keep him from "stimming" (doing repetitive meaningless motions, like pacing or using phrases over and over). "Do you love me?" might be cute the first time, but by the five hundredth time, it loses its charms. Although I'm not sure that watching television, which is pretty much what he chooses to do after work, is a fulfilling activity. He sings in the church choir, going to practice once a week, and goes to karate twice a week, where he's working on his black belt. On weekends, he and my husband like to do errands together on Saturdays (buying a pickle by himself at the farmer's market is a big hit) and go out to lunch. The three of us often go to the movies together, although we can also leave him home when we have a "date night" (no mushy romantic comedies, thank you), leaving the cell phone on vibrate. Sundays find us in church, where it is a huge pleasure for me to see him in the choir "blending in," albeit for one brief hour, followed by watching football on TV and yelling at the screen, which I have been assured is "normal adult male behavior." He cheers for all the Philadelphia teams, Phillies, Eagles, Flyers, often a hapless proposition. But he never gives up ("You can do it, boys!"). I can remember my mother being concerned for him when the Eagles lost in the Super Bowl. Instead, in David's World, the game was over, so he turned off the TV, and said "Next year." (Alas, we're still waiting. . . .)

We're also still waiting, for acceptance from the outside world. Hillary Clinton wrote how it takes a village to raise a child, but we've experienced social isolation, even shunning (like the Amish) in our journey. There was the playgroup I'd organized that he was asked to leave; ditto the baby-sitting cooperative. There were the "official" organizations in our area, Special Olympics, Make a Wish Foundation, Best Buddies, who all let us know that these groups were okay for children with Down syndrome, but children with autism need not apply. There were my in-laws, who first dismissed our concerns ("Oh, he's just got a little speech problem"—I guess not-speaking *would* qualify as a problem), then, after he received his diagnosis, stopped sending cards and gifts. It was as if he'd died, which in some ways, it was. One of my friends who worked in special education said we would be cycling through the five stages of grief over and over as we watched his contemporaries go to high school, get their licenses, marry, etc., while he remained the same, and she was right. When my oldest went off to college, I was in a parent seminar with people who were stressing over "what if my child picks the wrong major? Hates his or her roommate?" while I was worrying, "What if my other child ends up in an institution? Abused in foster care? Homeless?" The disparity between our lives and everyone else's is often huge.

So this is my world. Unlike my peers, who are enjoying their retirement by travelling the world via Elderhostel or going cross-country in an RV, I still need to arrange for childcare if I want to travel with my husband. Respite services are not available (many things "exist," they just aren't funded), so to do this, we have to find the right person (a responsible adult who's not working), train them, and write a document resembling a short Masters' thesis, giving instructions. Both of our adult daughters used to have Dave over for sleepovers, but they're in other states, with young families of their own now.

And there are other ways in which we are different: I was talking with a friend from college with a serious illness. She asked me, "What about you, how's your health?" I hadn't thought about this before, so I was hit by the realization that I *can't* get sick, because I'm the caregiver. Should, God forbid, one of us come down with, say, cancer, traveling out of the area to go to Johns Hopkins or the Mayo Clinic would be out of the question, because then who would watch David?

It's not all gloom and doom. I don't want to forget the pluses: Dave gives a mean back rub, has great thumbs. He's never reached the acting-out stage of adolescence, so he cheerfully mows the lawn in summer, hauls yard waste down the hill to our brush pile, shovels snow in winter, all huge helps for aging parents. He's the one (the only one?) in our church who puts money in an envelope each month for World Hunger; he watches the news with tears in his eyes. He answers the pastor's rhetorical questions and makes the congregation smile. He exemplifies "the pure in heart." My husband says he's here to teach us compassion and patience, two lessons I'm having to constantly re-learn. He faithfully watches *Wheel of Fortune* every night (an inexplicable favorite with ASD people) and Lawrence Welk re-runs every Saturday (also inexplicable).

And there've been unexpected bonuses, such as the use of our grandson as speech therapist. No one's ever sat down with him and said, "Your Uncle Dave has a disability," so Dan, at age six, has pretty much accepted Uncle Dave for who he is, although he's often puzzled by him. Once, when we were having dinner at their house, and realized we'd better be on the road as Dave had work the next day (they live two hours away).

"Work?" asked Dan. "But Uncle Dave's a kid. Kids don't work."

He and Dave like to watch *Sesame Street* (alas, Dan's aging out of that one, while Dave still loves it), listen to the Beatles, play with Legos (another of Dave's talents is his amazing ability to do Lego constructions, and also 3-D puzzles. His shining achievement has been to construct New York City, including rebuilding the World Trade Towers—all 3,266 pieces), etc. Dan has said, "I really love Uncle Dave, but he doesn't talk, does he?"

Talk about hitting the nail right smack on the head (Autism is considered largely a language and social impairment disorder). From that point on, Dan appointed himself Dave's "in your face" therapist, and he's been very persistent. Sometimes, all of the adults have been in one room, and we've realized, gosh, Dan and Dave are actually having a conversation, of sorts, in the other room.

One bit of grace is that Dave is far less "involved" (code word for "severity") than many of the children of our friends, who are virtual prisoners in their own lives, who can't leave their son or daughter alone, ever. And he's not violent; one of my friends had to place her son in a residential unit (that costs $100,000 a year, folks), as she feared for her life during his rage attacks. Nor does he have seizures. And his tics and quirks aren't severe enough to make us want to hide him at home, so we *can* go out in public to concerts, movies, train shows, etc. (Even though we sometimes get "the look," the one that implies, "Why isn't this person put away?")

But we're "aging out;" every day, it seems like new places ache that didn't before. I'm dealing with the fallout from an accident twenty years ago where I fractured my spine and tore my anterior cruciate ligament (caregivers with children who need to be driven to therapies can't have operations that requires six months of rehab and no driving). In this current political climate, where politicians self-righteously proclaim that it isn't right to tax the rich unless we cut "entitlement programs," (always said sneeringly; this means cutting what little help there is for people like David, who are not capable of taking care of themselves), I fall once again into existential despair. When I was caring for my dying mother (being a double-caregiver brings new meaning to the word "sandwich generation"), although it was difficult, especially emotionally, there was light at the end of the tunnel. And I knew that although I would miss her, this period of darkness we had entered would come to an end. With David, not only is there no light at the end of the tunnel, there's just the tunnel.

Someone in an upper tax bracket once asked me, "Why don't you just pay for a group home yourself?" (Underlying implication: "Why should WE pay for this?") The last time I looked, five years ago, the price tag was $40,000 a year, roughly the same as Assisted Living. We're looking at sixty years, most likely, a cool 2.4 million dollars. I don't know anyone who has this kind of money saved.

Another aspect of aging that preys on me constantly is, what if something happened to my husband? Right now, his providing transportation (and childcare when I travel) has freed me to live my writer's life, something I put on hold for many years. On icy winter mornings, because we live on top of a steep hill, I'd be afraid to drive David to work, and he'd probably lose his job. My husband and I each feel like we've each only been able to live half an adult life. But if (it's probably "when") I need to be a caregiver for my husband, how will I be able to take care of both of them? These are the things that keep me up at night.

In the end, I've been told by my social worker, "Don't die." I need to keep going forever. Oh, wait, that's impossible. And even more than the worry of will he have food, clean clothes, shelter, will he be protected from abuse, is the larger question, that when we're gone, who will love him?

And so I go on, pushing the stone (of his future) up the hill, daily. I know this is going to end badly, as we're likely to die first. But as the rabbi said in the Talmud, "It is not incumbent on your to finish the task. Neither are you free to give it up."

Parousia

Leslie Mahoney

"What I feared has come upon me;
what I dreaded has happened to me."
—Job 3:25

We are a bicoastal, bicultural, mutigenerational family. My youngest son, Dan, my daughter-in-law Jodi, and my grandchildren, Ruby and Harlan, live in Maine. My oldest son, Sean, my daughter-in-law, Diane and Diane's parents, Tess and Angel, live in Orange County, California. I live in a senior apartment not far from Sean and Diane.

During the annual family reunion in 2011, Dan took me aside and told me something was wrong with Sean—his walk was "off" and he couldn't coordinate his movements enough to run with Ruby and Harlan.

When I talked to Sean, he brushed it off saying he had forgotten how to run because he "didn't use this skill very often." I pushed for Sean to see his physician, but this didn't happen for several months. Sean's physician thought his "off" gait was work related and suggested physical therapy. The physical therapist asked Sean to jog down a hallway while dribbling an exercise ball. Sean couldn't coordinate his movements. The physical therapist wanted Sean seen by a neurologist.

When Sean told me, that horrible, dark, lonely place of fear opened deep inside of me. I know of this place; I have seen it on the face of others. Years of intensive care unit nursing taught me medical doublespeak. Sean's inability to coordinate his movements had nothing to do with a forgotten skill or his work. Something was very wrong.

The neurologist ordered MRIs—head, neck, spine and pelvis. Two weeks later, Sean called me and simply said, "Can you come over now?" The place of fear began to grow. As I drove to Sean's home, I repeated over and over—I will not react. I will be strong.

In the ICU, I had gentled families through fear, disbelief and loss with compassionate detachment. Now I was driving toward my own fear. The diagnosis was Multiple Sclerosis (MS).

Then came the spinal tap to confirm the diagnosis, the consultation with the MS specialist, and the six-month trial on Avonex.

We attended our first MS conference. The physician who spoke said he had been in MS research for 30 years and then decided to become a primary care physician for MS patients. He spoke about his years in research, which yielded no breakthroughs in the cause or cure for MS.

I had worked beside brilliant physicians. I had heard the evasions, the maybes, the medical jargon, the doublespeak when there were no answers. I had always accepted it until now. Now I wanted to scream. *How can you spend thirty years researching MS and not have answers? My son has MS—you have to have answers! Someone has to have answers!*

The fear inside me was surrounded by rage. My eyes stung as I held back the tears. I looked at Sean and Diane. They had questions. They went and talked with the physician. I already knew—the answers would be vague and inconclusive.

Sean began his own online research about MS. He became an MS "junkie"—online every night visiting MS chat rooms, reading articles about alternative therapy, and looking for new MS drug trials. He became involved in the MS community, the MS Walk-a-thon and co-editor of a collection of writings by people with MS to raise awareness about MS and money for MS research, *Something on Our Minds.*

The six-month trial on Avonex ended, and the repeat MRIs were done. The Avonex hadn't helped. There were new brain lesions. Now the diagnosis was more precise—Primary Progressive Multiple Sclerosis. The specialist hoped the progression would be slow.

Diane and Sean decided not to have children. Diane, at age thirty, is a child magnet! She can walk into a room full of children, and every child wants to be in her lap or cuddle with her. Her nephew Harlan has wanted to marry Diane since he was four. Diane and Sean had dreamed of having children, but now the MS had changed their dream.

We attended our second conference on "Diseases of the Brain." The physician was from New York University Medical Center. Aaron E. Miller, MD, FAAN spouted statistics like buckshot—MS drugs are incredibly expensive; MS drugs only work in 30% of the cases; we have no drugs that are effective for the progressive forms of MS; the few drug trials attempted with the progressive forms of MS exacerbated the disease.

I couldn't even feel the fear anymore. I couldn't feel the rage. I felt hollow, as if I had been gutted. Was this what Job felt? Where was hope? I had never, ever felt this way before in my entire life.

An image came back to me of the mother of a young man who died in the ICU after a terrible car accident. She came to see me three months after her son's death to talk about the nurses who cared for her son. The nurses were wonderful during her first visit to the ICU; they explained everything in great detail. But during each subsequent visit, this mother felt "pushed" to accept the inevitable—her son's injuries were too great, nothing would save his life. The mother knew in her head what her heart was not ready to accept. She had come to see me to implore the ICU staff not to destroy hope in the face of inevitable loss. She said her heart had needed time to live in hope for a little while longer.

I watch my son and daughter-in-law walking ahead of me. They walk holding hands, talking, looking at one another, laughing, nudging one another—perhaps oblivious to other people around them. Are they oblivious to what we just heard at the conference? How can they joke and laugh?

A few weeks after the conference, Sean and I go out to lunch. I slowly, haltingly bring up the conference. I ask the question I have been unable to answer. How do you and Diane come away from a conference like that, after hearing those statistics, and joke and laugh? I want to understand, how do you do that? Tell me, how you maintain hope?

Sean's demeanor changes. He becomes softer, gentler—like a mother nurturing a child. He says, "Yes, I have MS. But I live in today, this moment, right now, right here. In this moment, I am fine. Diane and I made a choice, a choice we make every day, that we will live in today; not in five years or ten years, but in each moment of each day." I nod my head to agree; I can't speak.

It has been two years since Sean was diagnosed with Multiple Sclerosis. I see the subtle physical change—the cautiousness on stairs, the wariness of uneven ground, the tiredness from walking, the unending sciatica that this disease brings. There are times when I must pull myself back from a dark place, a place of fear and pain and sorrow. In my mind, I repeat the wisdom of Emily Dickinson over and over:

> Hope is the thing with feathers
> That perches in the soul
> And sings the tune without the words
> And never stops
> at all.

I know the only way to deal with this fear is to walk through it— to feel it, to taste it, to be one with it, and to move on. This is not a one-shot deal. Each time I choose to walk through the fear, I can live in today. Today I can have lunch with Sean. I can feel the love we share. I hear "the tune without words" and know I am blessed.

Resource

Dickinson, Emily. "Hope Is the Thing with Feathers—(314)." *The Poetry Foundation*. The Poetry Foundation, 2013. Web. 20 Sept. 2013.

My Supposed Life

Alison Auerbach

This is not supposed to be my life. I am not supposed to be standing over a stove in my bathrobe and slippers, scrambling eggs at 7:40 on a Monday morning.

In the life I'm supposed to be living, the me that I planned to be is selecting a pair of shoes from her extensive funky footwear collection—something that will go with the casual, yet professional denim trousers she is wearing to work that day. Her children, Gabriel and Isabelle, are downstairs in the kitchen of our Cambridge townhouse, eating breakfast with this reality's version of my husband Ted. Since her first client arrives at the therapy office of the Boston Women's Health Collective earlier than his lecture starts at Harvard Medical School, he has breakfast with the kids and then helps them dress while she eats. Then she takes them to school via the T, Boston's public transportation system, and continues on to work, considering how to best disguise her clients' identities for her latest article.

Something is burning. While I've been creating pseudonyms for my nonexistent clients to use in my nonexistent article, a clot of scrambled egg has stuck to the frying pan and scorched. While I'm scraping it out, the microwave beeps, indicating that the bacon is done.

"My bacon, my bacon, my bacon!" chants Gabriel. "It's done! Can you get it? Please!"

"Dude! Please chill. I'm working as fast as I can here. It's coming, I promise."

I scrape the unburned scrambled egg and cheese onto a plate, slap the two slices of turkey bacon down next to it, add a couple of apple slices and garnish with half an anti-anxiety tablet. Then I slide the whole thing across the counter toward the top of my son's head. He's so intent on whatever iPhone game he is playing that his forehead is parallel to the floor. One hand pries itself off the phone and snags a piece of bacon off the plate.

"You're *welcome*."

"Thank you!" One hand sneaks toward the scrambled eggs.

"Use a fork! Please!" The hand veers off toward the fork.

Now I can eat. Back in Boston, the other me sips her coffee while skimming the *New York Times* headlines. After all, her husband is upstairs with the kids, so she has time to linger over her egg-white omelet and fruit salad. The burning-scrambled-eggs me has about three minutes to throw a half-cup of yogurt, a drizzle of honey, and a scoop of frozen fruit into the cup of the immersion blender. Today turns out to be one of the frequent occasions on which I turn the blender on before it's fully immersed in the yogurt. Now it's also a facial.

"Mom! Come play Cut the Rope with me!"

"Let me just finish getting my breakfast together, Big Shot. I'll be right there."

"But it's already 7:52!" Despite his anti-anxiety medication, Gabriel still tends to fixate on the time. He knows his morning routine down to the minute, and he becomes agitated if he believes he is falling behind. It's hard for me to help him overcome this, because I empathize.

I too love schedules and order. The difference is that I don't cry or have a panic attack if we leave the house at 8:41 instead of 8:40. Then again, the world isn't a constant unpredictable assault of sensory input on my nervous system, as it is for Gabriel, so I am somewhat less dependent on routines as a way to help me navigate my surroundings. His medication has taken enough of the edge off that he doesn't melt down completely with slight variations in his routine. But he is still very clock-conscious.

So though it goes against every instinct I have to leave the dirty blender and coffee pot in the sink to wash later, our morning ritual must go on as scheduled. While the other me is washing out the coffee pot in her antique farmhouse sink, I am blotting yogurt off my eyebrows as I sit down to play Cut the Rope with my son.

The object of Cut the Rope, an iPhone/iPad game, is to feed a piece of candy to a small green beast named Om Nom (after his munching sound). On each level, the candy is suspended from various configurations of ropes, floating in bubbles, dangling over spikes and so on. There are three stars on each level, and the more of them the candy hits on the way to Om Nom, the more points you get. The player cuts the ropes, pops the bubbles, and so forth to get the candy directly into Om Nom's mouth, as the little bugger is apparently unable to lift a paw to grab the thing out of the air, even if it's dangling right next to him.

No morning is complete without a few rounds of Cut the Rope—for both of us. It's not enough for Gabriel to play the game while he eats breakfast. I have to be sitting next to him, playing the game on my iPad while he plays it on the iPhone. We have to start on the exact same level at the exact same time. When Om Nom eats the candy, one of us must say "Yum, yum!" and the other one must answer "Yum, yum, yum, yum!" Then we compare scores.

His is always higher.

Our mutual worship at the Altar of Om Nom is one of a handful of mentally organizing activities that Gabriel uses to gear up for the demands of his day. I respect the need for a child's routine to include such activities, and so does the other me. That's why she reads aloud to Gabriel and Isabelle on the T on the way to school each day. And none of the old favorites she shares with her children include a lazy, green, candy-scarfing beast.

As I have no client expecting me, I am determinedly yanking on gym clothes. I missed yesterday's workout for an auction committee meeting at Gabriel's school. Somehow, I, the girl who dreaded group projects from kindergarten through graduate school, am co-chairing this annual fundraising event. Today, I am going to make time for this workout, mostly to relieve some of my mounting guilt.

After dropping Gabriel at school, I head to the YMCA for an hour on the elliptical trainer. I hate exercise. However, I do reluctantly recognize that it reduces my stress level as much as three glasses of wine, but with fewer side effects. It also allows me to watch *Charmed*, a teen soap that somehow managed to combine *Charlie's Angels* with *Buffy the Vampire Slayer* and retained the merits of neither. If demons were real, and I was going to fight them, I would not be wearing a tube top. And I most certainly would be wearing a bra. Today's episode is the one where good-witch Phoebe Halliwell discovers that the man with whom she has fallen in love is actually a demon. I love this one.

The other me fits in her exercise on the days she works from home. She uses the facilities at Harvard, thanks to her Ted's faculty status. She might multitask on the elliptical trainer by listening to recorded books or take a Yoga or dance class for a change of pace. If she did happen to watch *Charmed*, it would probably be research for a media studies article.

By the time I reach my cool down, Phoebe has convinced her sister witches that she has vanquished the love of her life (even though she couldn't bring herself to kill him and let him escape into hiding). Since TNT cycles through all seven years' worth of *Charmed* about every four months, I know that she will live to regret this choice. And I allow myself a mental "you'll be sorry" as I wipe down the elliptical for the next user. It's weirdly satisfying to know better than this lovely, fashionable, brave, intelligent and entirely fictional woman.

Once I'm home, I grab my receipt file and head for the computer. It's Thursday, so my daily household task is to handle the finances. This includes entering all checks, electronic payments and ATM withdrawals into a computerized register; checking the credit card company's transaction record for the week against our receipts; filing the receipts; balancing the checkbook as necessary and paying bills. Our financial planner thinks that doing all of this each week is a bit excessive, but we've agreed to disagree on that point.

Gabriel has Om Nom. I have my to-do list. In fact, I have it with me all the time, as it's stored in my phone. It's divided into six, color-coded categories, from which the program creates a daily list based on the due date for each task. Weekly tasks, like my finance update, are set to repeat on assigned days. On Monday, grocery shopping pops up on the list. On Tuesday, it's filing and paperwork. Wednesday is laundry day, and Thursday is, of course, finance day.

Up in Boston, the other me has figured out how to automate the entire financial update process. She doesn't plan menus or spend much time in the grocery store, as her local CSA delivers most of the produce her family needs. Gabriel and Isabelle consider it a treat to be allowed to help their dad invent that night's dinner, for which he is always home. The other me might take care of a little filing while they cook, but she's got the household almost entirely paperless, so there isn't much to file. But I bet she still has a to-do list, even though most of the household tasks are on autopilot. Some things will be a part of my life in any reality.

I have always been frighteningly organized, a little too fond of storage bins and unnaturally attached to my label maker. The unpredictability of motherhood, particularly special-needs motherhood, simply ramped up my existing need for control over my surroundings. That little adrena-line shot transformed my once-humble to-do list into the color-coded, categorized beast of today. It also fed my obsession with labels of all kinds—not just the sticky-backed variety, but also the invisible kind.

Homemaker. Stay-At-Home-Mom (or, in the Internet chat room age, SAHM). Domestic Engineer. Executive Household Manager. Family CEO. Housewife.

Though I hate every one of these labels, a lack of better alternatives has forced me to use most of them at least once since deciding to give up gainful employment to care for my son. My dad, a highly experienced CPA, does our taxes and persists in listing my occupation as "homemaker," despite repeated requests to change it to "social worker" (which reflects my graduate degree) or "case manager" (which better reflects the work I do on behalf of my son). To a man of his generation, a married woman with a child who does not hold a full-time paying job is a homemaker.

Thanks to women like Martha Stewart and Rachel Ray (who I respect as successful businesswomen in their own right), the term homemaker now brings to mind a woman who changes her living room decor to match the season, cans vegetables from her heirloom-seeded garden, and hand sews her children's Halloween costumes. I don't mean to suggest that there's anything wrong with any of these tasks or with the desire to do them. But I don't have that desire, and I don't do those things.

"Domestic Engineer" and "Executive Household Manager" are so politically correct that they make even me gag, me—a feminist so far left that I'm practically falling off the continuum. They smack of desperation, of the need to justify the decision to work hard for no pay. As though full-time home management is a luxury that has to be justified, and not a heart-rending choice influenced by the flexibility of one's job, one's spouse's job, financial need, the availability of decent child care and health care, one's personal definition of what it means to be a good mother and a thousand other things. As though it's always a decision based on personal preference.

The label Stay-At-Home-Mom is popularly used to describe a woman whose full-time (unpaid) occupation is mothering, rather than paid employment away from home. When I hear it, I can't help thinking that it sounds like I'm not allowed to leave the house. Does my son need a second mom for travel? And do I need some sort of permit to go out with my husband? My reality is that I'm rarely physically present in my home during working hours, and since Gabriel is in school full time, the largest chunk of my day is not spent actively mothering.

The other me doesn't have to choose among these labels that don't describe her at all. And that's perhaps the most difficult to swallow of the differences between the life I'm living and the life I'm supposed to be living. We use our job titles as social shorthand for who we are. The other me has a job title and a professional identity not tied to her children, her husband, or her home: She's a therapist. My job has no appropriate title (SAHM-feminist-social-worker-advocate-community-volunteer doesn't really roll off the tongue) and my work barely qualifies as a profession by today's standards. My identity, as separate from Gabriel, Ted, and my home, remains ambiguous and ill-defined. To me, and everyone else.

Ambiguous and ill-defined! Me, the woman with the to-do list on steroids. The missing label is unsettling, to say the least. The life I was supposed to be living is orderly and contained, everything in the right place, running on schedule. The life I'm living is...messy. There's yogurt in my eyebrows for God's sake.

If my life was a Hollywood film, this would be the part where I'm supposed to confess that I've embraced the chaos and enjoy the freedom of living without labels. If my life was a Hollywood film, I would look like Halle Berry instead of like me. Neither of those things is going to happen anytime soon. My reality is that my discomfort with my life's messiness is as much a part of me as the face in the mirror and is more difficult to change (though I admit that even the very best plastic surgeon would find it challenging to make me look like Halle Berry).

Eventually, I suppose, my recalcitrant identity and I will reach some sort of cease-fire, if not an actual truce. I'll stop trying to shoehorn it into perfect little boxes if it will stop working so hard to defy definition. In the meantime, I take comfort in the knowledge that at least one other person in my life understands the beauty of order.

After I alphabetized our collection of 50 or so spices in matching, labeled tins (a project that took me the better part of two days), Gabriel gazed in awe at the finished display.

"Look how pretty it is!" he whispered.

I couldn't agree more.

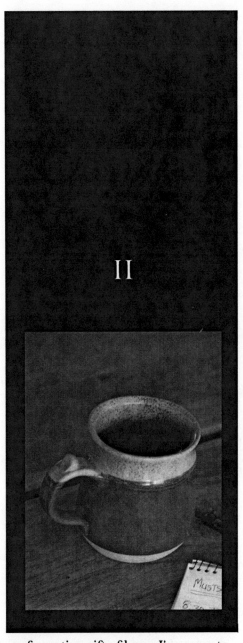

II

"And through the transformative gift of hope, I've come to believe in my blood and in my bones that my son will continue to grow, that his bud will open and reveal a beauty so extraordinary that its power will transform our lives. Indeed, he already has."
-Jennifer Meade

When Life Gave Me Lemons, A Pie Was My Weapon

Julie Mairano

When life gave me lemons, a pie was my weapon. It wasn't always this way.

Lisa's life demanded twenty-four seven care and was always a challenge for us. The same people who were supposed to help us often shied away. Only four-feet tall and weighing forty-eight pounds, she was twelve years old and could neither walk nor talk. As painful as it was to watch other's reaction to her small size, her missing ring finger, and her unusual facial features, when I saw her through my husband's eyes she was beautiful. His oldest daughter, my husband the builder, called her his very own "four by four!"

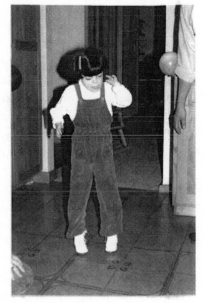

With no survival instincts, her safety demanded a house with no knickknacks to shatter, lamps to tip over, or small pieces to swallow. Friends soon learned if they were not watchful of where they placed their drinks, Lisa would do her best to drink them for them.

Yet, hope was always present that her life would be better and any milestone (a babble, learning to drink from a cup, or mastering the sign for drink) was celebrated. But none as much as when her school called to say she had taken her first steps.

"We're all crying here but not because we have sad news. I want to tell you great news, so you can plan a celebration. Lisa took two steps today." It was the day before her twelfth birthday, and family and friends were called and asked to join us the next night rather than wait for her scheduled birthday party on Sunday. We had a big surprise!

What we had forgotten was that Lisa often tested our patience, and this day would be no different. Dressed in her denim coveralls and white Peter Pan collared blouse, Lisa greeted her guests by holding each hand for a minute, carefully detecting if there was any trace of

81

medical smell and assuring herself that this was a person she could trust. Her guests knew how to greet her, offering their hands and waiting patiently until she took their hand and held it in hers.

Dinner finished, Lisa sat on her special chair, making her sign for dessert, mini-marshmallows. One by one, each guest approached her, mini-marshmallows held only a few steps out of her reach, hoping she would choose to reach out to them and take a step. But they were rewarded only with a smirk of a smile and a refusal to place either foot on the floor. I knew this child liked to test my patience; I was reminded that she had also taught me the value of persistence. Armed with only hope, I picked her up, carried her upstairs, tucked her in bed and proceeded to invite everyone for a second birthday celebration for the next day.

The sun greeted me brightly the next morning as I carried Lisa to the special education van and asked her driver to let her sleep on the way home so that she would be rested for her second party. Once again, family and friends arrived as Lisa finished her dinner, but this time I had a plan. Placing a pile of mini-marshmallows in her direct line of site but a full two steps away, I watched and waited as she looked at each of us and made the sign for food and was ignored by all. Time slowed, and with it, we all grew weary and disappointed believing that this night would be no different then the last and turned our attention to enjoying the left-over birthday cake. Would Lisa understand that if she wanted marshmallows she would need to get them herself?

Silence, then tears slowly filled the room as one by one we became aware that she had quietly slid off her chair, taken two steps, and was grabbing the marshmallows and stuffing them in her mouth and continued her journey into the family room with all the assurance of someone who had practiced this for years. Being once again the center of attention, she continued her journey into the family room with all the assurance of someone who had practiced walking for years. The applause was deafening as she gave a big grin to all her teary eyes fans who knew that a miracle had occurred. No longer would Lisa always have to depend on others to go where she wanted to go. Toasts were made and champagne flowed freely until everyone was too tired to laugh or cry.

The following Sunday afternoon, however, we received an un-expected home visit from her geneticist, the doctor who had diagnosed her with Cornelia de Lange Syndrome (CdLS). He had also been trained as a pediatrician and had offered to help us find one for her, but with much persuading, he soon agreed to accept Lisa as his only pediatric patient. Like us, he wished for a better life for Lisa and was closely invested in helping her reach her full potential. He had been with us since her birth, taking midnight phone calls and meeting us at the emergency room but had never visited our home. He had last seen her the week before her birthday for her annual check-up and had sent us for a full set of X-rays hoping to discover why she was not walking. He had been away for the past week and not able to attend the party, and I was sure he had come to see her walking firsthand and join in the celebration.

The car stopped at the top of our driveway, and we watched as he slowly came our way. His voice was gentle; his words were not. He had come to tell us that the X-ray report showed Lisa's femurs needing immediate attention. Unless she had an operation, her walking would be short-lived. Her stay in the hospital would be a long one.

I reached for my husband and held on; my joyful time had passed so quickly. Once again, my husband would become full-time caretaker of our other two children. Even though I would insist that she be cared for like any other child, those that knew her soon learned that Lisa was not like most children. Her veins were tiny, her energy unlimited, and her stubbornness legendary. Body boards did not her contain her, and all were afraid that her arm would break before she held still enough for a blood sample. She did not talk but knew how to control her world and often made poor decisions such as refusing to drink water unless she was outside the walls of the hospital, necessitating long stroller rides no matter what the weather. Stories of her strength and her ability to foil even the best-laid plans of seasoned doctors filled her medical files. Both nurses and doctors depended on my mother's instincts to guide them with Lisa's care.

The decision was made that evening. Without the surgery, she could lose the ability to walk forever. How could we deny her the operation? I knew the risks of anesthesia and long hospital stays, but I had also spent every Thursday morning with her working with physical therapists who were making her strong enough to walk. How could I give up now?

Two weeks later, I drove to the Children's Hospital and entered "our" room. Piled high with books and clothing that would protect my decency when doctors arrived at all hours, I wept for the unknown and the not-knowing if this trip would be her last. No one knew how long children with CdLS might live. Was I tempting fate by being so aggressive with her care? Did I want too much for her?

Days and weeks passed slowly. The surgery went well, but her recovery was more complicated then expected. Bound in a body cast, she had begun to have fevers and was refusing to eat. It took weeks before she was diagnosed with acid reflux, given medication and was back on the road to recovery. My husband and my children joined me for dinner every Saturday and "our" little room took on a life of its own. Inside I created a small office, my home computer perched on the windowsill, a printer tucked under her empty bed, and a file drawer on her nightstand. In this way, I was able to continue corresponding with others who were also caring for children with her syndrome, hoping that someone knew more than I about her condition. Phone calls, however, were expensive, and the isolation that came with the closed door grew as the days passed.

Fall was coming to a close, and as I searched the TV channels trying to find any escape from my thoughts that soon even outside walks with Lisa in the stroller would be impossible, there was a knock on my door. It was hours past visiting time, but there she stood, my Cher-like coworker from my days spent at the Department of Children and Family Services reminding me of my past life—a life before Lisa.

Her tears streamed as she approached me with a Kleenex in one hand and a large white box, neatly wrapped in baker's string with the other. She had learned that although the hip surgery appeared to have gone well, Lisa's recovery was difficult and long and said ever so quietly, "I thought you might need this?" Laura, who never travelled alone because of her fear her abusive ex-husband might find her, had risked her well being to take care of me.

I knew by her smile that something good had to be inside this box. Having survived on hospital food for more weeks than I cared to remember, I slowly untied the thin, white string to discover a pie shell, piled high with soft, cloud-like meringue perched on top of four inches of bright lemon filling. There was only one fork. Presented with this opportunity, I broke all the rules about sharing and inhaled the sweet smell of the lemons, teased the meringue until it stood tall on each forkful and ate every morsel until all that remained was a metal pie pan, with the words twenty-five cent deposit imprinted on the bottom.

Within moments, the sugar high began, and my feelings of isolation and hopelessness disappeared. I knew that bad things could change your life in a moment. I had forgotten that good things could change your life too. Without sadness, you would not know true joy. The weekly pie visits soon became a ritual that included the arrival of a Snoopy lunchbox with a gift for Lisa and a matching thermos filled with

Pinot Grigio wine for me. Her visits became a forever reminder that there are good things in this world if we look for them.

The hospital staff looked forward to these "way past visiting hours" arrivals of Laura as much as Lisa and I did. They could see the smile on my face brighten or the sadness in my eyes lessen when she arrived, and they kindly looked the other way as we propped Lisa in a stroller or carried her and explored the empty ghost white hallways and forbidden operating areas. We walked, we talked, and most of all we laughed as I shared all the silly ways the doctors and nurses had tried to bribe Lisa into cooperating. We knew better than to let other parents who were staying at the hospital know of our late night travels. We dared not ask permission lest we lose our privileges.

Lemon meringue pies kept arriving, and my purpose in life grew clearer. If I were to help Lisa, I would need to share her story not only with other families, but also with professionals who could make a difference. And so our hospital room became grand central for in-service lectures for anyone interested in learning more about CdLS and the grass-roots organization that was forming to provide help and hope for children like her.

Fast forward through my life, and you will see Lisa and me sharing a hospital room many more times and being visited by Laura, my family, or friends. Laura would always arrive with a lemon meringue pie and one fork and remind me that Lisa's greatest joy was walking. I'd half-laughing share that now she would sit down only when it was time to eat or sleep.

Last year, twenty-two years after Laura's first visit, Lisa and I took her final trip to the hospital. Her body was failing, and she was in pain; there was little we could do except let her know how much we loved her and make her as comfortable as possible. Family and friends came to say goodbye and celebrate the ways she inspired them and others to be better people. They came with love; they came with food. There was no need for pie.

Whatever It Takes
Claudia Malacrida

My beautiful daughter. Straight back, round head, sweet, smart, beanie. Standing at the bus stop every morning, amid happy, laughing children. Going to school, eager to learn, eager to live, eager to be part of it all. She is seven years old.

It is a lovely winter morning—crisp and sunny and glistening. I strip the duvet off the bed and lay it on the open windowsill to air. Pausing, I breathe in the delights of the day—dazzling sunlight, sparkling snowdrifts, the chirp and flutter of myriad small birds, and—slowly it comes to me—the sound of children's voices. Chanting.

"We hate Hilary! We hate Hilary! We hate Hilary!"

I strain to hear. I'm not wrong, I *do* hear it—"We hate Hilary! We hate Hilary!"

Running, wearing only slacks and a shirt, I cover the distance to the bus stop. Heart pounding, voice quaking, I address this gaggle of four-foot tall torturers, speak to their better nature, beg for their compassion, appeal to their shame. Sullen. The silence is deadening.

The bright yellow bus rounds the corner, pulls up, its door swinging open. Two by two, the children board the bus. My daughter, my beautiful, brave daughter, gets on as well, to be taken off to a place I now no longer believe is either innocent or safe.

*

And so it began. The first inkling—no, that's not true—the first confirmation that something terribly bad was happening to my beautiful girl. After all, that nagging worry was what led me to volunteer in the classroom and take a job working lunch hours as a playground supervisor. So I could keep an eye on things.

But that incident at the bus stop crystallized my doubts. I could no longer deny that she was slowly, almost imperceptibly drifting away from me, that she was no longer her curious, happy self. From that moment forward, I could never again assume that for Hilary things are okay or that the world in which she lives is safe.

That night, until very late in the night, my husband and I talk. We talk about how our plan to remain in student family housing while I finish my degree might have to change. We talk about how we might have to switch our daughter's school. We talk about how scared we are for her. We acknowledge our lack of power to protect her and our confusion over why this is happening to someone who we know is simply, wonderfully, lovable. We mourn our innocence, our dream that she would steer the shoals of childhood unharmed.

No—that's not true—I talk, while my husband listens quietly, unsure whether my dark view is necessarily right. He is less dark than I am. But still, he knows this is serious, and he listens with sad, if grudging, respect.

*

The next day, I meet the school principal, her classroom teachers, the vice principal. I tell them of our concerns: that Hilary is an outcast, that she seems unhappy, that sometimes she doesn't want to go to school. They tell me they have no concerns whatsoever. Hilary is a good girl, no bother in the classroom. And no, there haven't been problems at this school with bullying, but they promise to keep an eye on things.

I leave that meeting uncomforted. Instead, I feel that the people to whom I have consigned my daughter's care have neither the will nor the ability to truly rise to the occasion. I feel that my words have not been heard, that my daughters' problems have not been understood, and that nothing—nothing—is going improve. I feel lonely, angry and scared. Lonely, because it seems that I am the only one who can see that this is a serious thing. Angry, because my complaints have been responded to as though I were hysterical. And scared because I am beginning to realize that I am going to have to find a way out of this, and I have no map.

*

Despite my education and my experience and my passionate concern, I don't know what to do. I try to talk with Hilary, and she's like a locked box. She won't talk, she doesn't answer. And I worry that by prying, I am placing yet one more pressure on her already burdened small shoulders.

I talk obliquely. I bring up conversations about her school in what I hope will be casual ways. I volunteer in the schoolyard and watch for the bullies, for the bad kids. They aren't obvious. What is obvious, however, is that my daughter, who I think is funny and smart and full of life, is almost always alone at school. What is also obvious is that the children look at me with more than a little hostility. It's as though we're somehow marked, my daughter and I. We are different and thus, suspect.

*

Hilary speaks, finally. She says, "Can I change schools?"

This is not a question that I find difficult to take in. I have, after all, seen firsthand what her life is like in that school. But there is more than just this knowledge that propels my acceptance, and it has as much to do with my own history as my love for my daughter. I find that more and more I am drawn back to my own childhood, and to the memories of being a child who was "different." I am flooded with the memories of my own childish inability—despite fervent intentions—to understand what was going on in the classroom, to "be good," to belong. I remember the taunting, the isolation, and the prayers that, with each new school year, were a mantra:

> This time it will be different. This time I will keep my math book looking neat and tidy. This time I will not lose my gloves, or spend recess in the hallway because I have forgotten to bring my science project to school. This time the teacher will like me, and I will be popular. This time, this time.

I also remember with bitterness the teachers, who called me lazy or a liar or who simply said "could do better." I remember, too, the extra burden of having a mother who seemed to be disappointed and humiliated by me. And in my remembering, I find some resolve. I resolve that I will never do that to Hilary, that I will always let her know that I love her, and that I have her back. So, when she asks for a new chance at a new school, I say, "Yes. Whatever it takes."

*

My husband and I talk again, and in one late night epiphany decide that we can buy a house, that we can do this. I know then that I am blessed, that although I might be the woman with the dark vision and emotional baggage, I am not going to fight alone. I have my partner, my wonderful partner, who understands and agrees that the most important thing we can do is "whatever it takes."

Within two days, we buy a modest house we can barely afford, and I take Hilary to visit her new school.

It's charming. Small. Traditional-style classrooms. Unlike her present school with its open plan and team teaching. There is artwork on the walls, and the hallways smell of wax, and Hilary slips her hand inside mine and tells me, "This school feels safe, Mom."

I feel a crack open in my chest, and fight hard not to cry. I don't want to cry in front of her. I don't want her to see that I am worried. I don't want her to know how sorry I am that she should have to say such a hard thing at such a young age. I don't want her to understand that I haven't got the answers, only more questions. At least for today, I want her to believe in safety, and yes—part of me wants to believe in it myself.

I decide she shouldn't wait until we have moved before she starts her new school. I just want it to be okay, and the sooner the better. I rearrange my class schedule and drive her to and from the new school.

I say, "Whatever it takes."

*

Now that she's at the new school, Hilary begins to tell us about the harassment she has suffered, the name-calling, the ostracism. I guess she feels she can tell us this, now she knows she's never going back.

At the old school, I attend an exit interview. I sit in the little chair at the table, while the teacher sits in an adult chair across from me. I know about the power relations embedded in this seating arrangement, but I can't quite bring myself to stand up and suggest we sit on the sofa at the back of the room. Besides, how bad can this be? I am, after all, only here to pick up her books.

The teacher is a woman who only speaks to me with her eyes closed. I never learn what color they are. In the intervening years, however, I have imagined them grey and flat.

She hands me Hilary's report card. It is glowing. Hilary is bright, hardworking, and achieving well, it says. I am given the work she has accomplished during the first seven months of the school year. The contents fit inside a small envelope. She has done nothing for seven months.

In this moment, I begin to understand the chasm that separates the written record of Hilary's school life and the actual experiences of her education. I begin to understand that nobody is willing to tell the truth on paper—not if it means that they might be held responsible. I begin to understand that we do not share the same priorities when it comes to my daughter. As I begin to understand these things, I feel something old and angry rising up in me.

I decide not to be polite. I decide not to take the package and just disappear. I decide instead to tell the teacher about how my daughter has not wanted to come to school, that she sometimes pretends illness so that she can stay home. I tell her about the harassment. About the little boy who bullied her, whose language and behavior, had they not come from a seven-year-old, would have been termed sexual harassment. The teacher, through closed lids, says, "Oh. That explains it then."

I say, "Explains what?"

She replies, "Well, I always suspected that Hilary might be sexually abused."

I say nothing. I am so angry, so stunned, so outraged that I cannot put my thoughts into words. I wonder why, if she had really thought that my daughter was at risk, she hadn't bothered to do anything about it. I wonder what she must think about me, and my husband, and our home. I wonder what kind of comments and concerns she might have included in our file—the one that will precede my daughter to her new school.

I wonder, and rage, and say nothing. I am cowed and leave quietly, with the small envelope of schoolwork crushed in my fingers. I unlock the car door and sit, holding the steering wheel for a long time before I drive home.

*

It's better here at the new school. The Grade Two classroom has rows of desks, the teacher is firm and organized, and Hilary has made a couple of tentative friends within weeks. However, the teacher pulls me aside and says, "We have to talk."

It seems that Hilary is so far behind in her schoolwork that they think she might need to repeat Grade Two. I know enough to understand that failing a grade will not be good, especially since she's had some social problems already. I make a deal with the teacher.

"Give me time," I say, "we'll get her caught up."

I take her to a tutor for Math, and we send her to summer school, so she can catch up on her writing and reading. We try to make it seem like a treat—she is going to go to a special class and will have lots of fun, and it will be in the big high school up the road—the high school she will someday attend. Won't that be grown up?

Hilary is a peach. She thrives on the individual attention and catches up on her work at a level that astounds everyone but me and my husband. We know she is smart. We begin to wonder why they can't see it.

During this summer, I am taking two courses so I can finish my degree quickly. I change the classes I will take so that I can fit my schedule around the summer school. I also take a part-time job to help defray the costs of the summer school.

"Oh well," I say. "Whatever it takes."

*

Whatever it has taken has, in the intervening years, proved to be quite considerable. Further, it has never been clear, in the moment, exactly what it *should* take to do the right thing. This lack of certainty, and my resulting lack of confidence, has been a constant challenge. Am I doing the right thing? Am I overreacting? Is this a person I can trust? Is this really an improvement?

In Grade Three, her teacher still could not seem to reach her and called me endlessly, saying:

> "Hilary is not doing well in Math. Is there something wrong at home?"
> "Hilary's homework has not been done. Is there something wrong at home?"
> "Hilary's agenda has not been signed. Is there something wrong at home?"
> "Hilary does cartwheels in the cloakroom. Is there something wrong at home?"
> "Hilary doesn't seem able to connect with her peers. Is there something wrong at home?"

By now, my husband and I are doing upwards of two hours of homework a night with Hilary. No longer are we playing catch-up because of the first school. Now we are playing catch-up because Hilary is struggling at this school. By the end of each night's homework session, Hilary and I are usually both crying. I feel resentment about the amount of time I am spending teaching my child what she didn't learn in the daytime and about the homework fights that I don't feel are rightly mine. I begin to think that maybe this problem should belong to her teachers instead.

Finally, her teacher calls and I say, "No. There is nothing wrong at home. It's time we asked what is wrong at school."

She isn't impressed, but I am tired, I am pissed, and I am no longer willing to placate this woman. I don't think she's worth it. I don't care whether she thinks I'm a nice mother. More importantly—I don't think that all my efforts at being nice have done my daughter much good. Sometimes "whatever it takes" is surprising. Sometimes "whatever it takes" means saying no.

Thus begins a round of meetings that culminate in one memorable one. Sitting in the principals' office—on one side, the two classroom teachers, the school's resource teacher, the school psychologist, the vice principal, the principal and the school board's program specialist—on the other, my husband and I.

As I sit in this meeting, no longer a child, but an adult with more education and more intimate knowledge of my child than anyone else in the room, I find myself taken back to similar meetings in which I sat staring at the floor while teachers and principals told my mother that I was impossible, and my mother wept. Meetings where I understood completely what was going on, but never had the ability to speak out and be heard. Meetings where my chest burned with anger and frustration and shame when adult eyes would turn to me and ask me, "Why *can't* you...?"

It was always the question I never knew the answer to.

Hilary does not attend this meeting, so at the very least she does not have to watch *me* crying as I sit in that room full of strangers. Even though I am crying, I do not believe my child is impossible. I do not believe that she needs fixing. Instead, I believe there is something wrong with her teachers. They may be nice enough women, but they are not doing what they say they are doing—they are not teaching her. I know this—because I have gone over the subtraction tables with Hilary for three years now, and she still cannot understand them. I know this, because I go over her spelling with her every week, and she continues to make the same mistakes. I know this, because she is—again—drifting away from us. And so I push for answers, I ask for suggestions, I ask for help. And I refuse blame—for Hilary or for our family.

In this meeting, for the first time, someone says the words "Attention Deficit Disorder" and asks us to consider Ritalin. She has not yet been tested, but they know the solution.

This is where things really get rough for me. I think of all the things I've read about ADD, and all the claims that it's just another diagnosis used to keep children docile. Zombies, the articles say. Kiddie cocaine. Children drugged because teachers can no longer maintain discipline.

I think of all the things I've read about psychiatry and psychology. That the number of categories for psychiatric disorders has tripled in the past twenty years. That, once a category like ADD is made to exist, with all its vague symptoms, and its lack of a "hard" test for diagnosing, it becomes very easy—too easy—to apply the label. That the rates of diagnosis and medication have skyrocketed, particularly since education cuts have come into vogue.

I think of all the times that I, as a young child, was the focus. How everyone—educators, doctors and psychologists alike—presumed that I was the problem and never asked about the teacher or the school or my classmates.

I think of all this and I agree—reluctantly, grudgingly, achingly—to an assessment. I am desperate. Despite my doubts, I must do something, anything, if it will help. I square my shoulders, and I say, "Whatever it takes."

*

And so begins a long investigation into services for children suspected of ADD in our area. The options are endless, as are the numbers of specialists. A multi-modal assessment is the ideal procedure, according to the private agencies that offer them. Their fees are astronomical. The Children's Hospital has a one-year waiting list for multi-modal assessments covered by public health care. The pediatricians specializing in ADD all have six-month waiting lists.

Finally, we see a pediatrician. Twenty minutes later, we leave her office with one Xeroxed sheet of questions and a prescription for a double-blind Ritalin test. The pills are split between Ritalin and placebos. We and the teacher are each to complete a daily questionnaire, which I will bring back to the Doctor for assessment.

I read the questionnaire—it asks about the ability to sit still, take turns, stand in line, work in groups. There is nothing about her life outside the classroom—at home, on the playground, with peers. The first pill that I give her catapults our stolid, easygoing child into a panic attack while shopping, and we have to take her home. There is no place on the form for me to provide this information.

The teacher fills out her forms assiduously—a neat row of X's that easily relate to Hilary's classroom experiences. I add commentary and concerns—my forms look like examination crib notes. When I give both stacks to the pediatrician, she carefully removes those that I completed, telling me that because school behavior is the problem, those won't be necessary. She quickly looks at the columns, checks Hilary's weight and writes a prescription. I fill it at the pharmacy, because I have no idea what else to do.

I am not pleased. I am not relieved. I am not convinced. I don't feel that—yes, finally—here is the answer. Instead, this diagnosis—and the treatment—seems too easy.

I've taken books from the library and surfed the web. I've called support groups and spoken to other parents. I've attended workshops and spoken with people at special clinics and medical offices. I have found out as much as I can about ADD. And even though I recognize my daughter in a great deal of the literature, the "symptoms" seem so natural to childhood that I have a hard time accepting this is as a "disorder."

Also, much of the information is conflicting. ADD is a modern malaise, engineered by teachers and psychologists who cannot teach. ADD is a modern malaise, engineered by parents—mostly mothers—who are too lazy or too selfish or too busy to parent properly. ADD is the result of not being breastfed and should be treated with vitamins. ADD stems from stressful lifestyles and is usually the result of family dysfunction, or—gasp—working mothers who cannot provide the kind of attention children really need. ADD is caused by junk food and poor diet. ADD can be treated through massage, biofeedback, whole food diets, essential fatty acid supplements, counseling, self-esteem workshops, all of which cost, and none of which seem convincing.

And so I begin, each morning, to place two small blue pills next to her plate. Despite her constant stomachache. Despite the teacher's continued complaints about her organizational problems. Despite the ongoing grind of ever-increasing homework. Despite my own ambivalence. I can think of no alternative, and as I place the pills next to her plate each day, I say, "Whatever it takes."

*

Hilary continues to take Ritalin. She also continues to bring home homework that inexorably erodes our family's relationships. We work each night for two or three hours, my husband and I taking turns, as each of us reaches the point of no return. Hilary has no option—she has no one to spell her off. It is terrible, terrible, terrible. She cries, I cry.

94

We go to bed sometimes at ten at night, without kissing goodnight, grateful that we need not endure any more for that night.

She regularly misses Girl Guides. She does not ever miss her regular private Math tutoring. We are all doing whatever we can to make this work, and we are failing, failing.

Still, the phone calls from the teacher:

> "Hilary is not doing well in Math class. Is there
> something wrong at home?"
> "Hilary's homework has not been done. Is there
> something wrong at home?"
> "Hilary's agenda has not been signed. Is there
> something wrong at home?"
> "Hilary doesn't seem able to connect with her
> peers. Is there something wrong at home?"

Yes, there is. I am worried sick for our lovely, struggling, quiet, uncomplaining, slowly fading away daughter.

＊

End of Grade Three. Hilary is going to go into a special classroom for children with Learning Disabilities. The school says, "This is a Good Thing. We take special care to ensure that children are integrated with the rest of the school. She will still be able to be with her friends. She will take some subjects in the regular class, and do English, Math, Science, and Social Studies in the LD class. We've seen this before, and we know. It's what she needs."

We hope. We trust. Even though we have been given little reason to, we trust. Despite my concerns about "special placements," we sign the form.

I think, "Well, maybe this is the answer."

I say, "Whatever it takes."

＊

For the next two years, Hilary attends this special class. I volunteer several days a week, helping children read, keeping peace in the library. I am not a teacher, but I sometimes wonder whether this class is such a good thing. Granted, there are only twelve children for the one teacher, but they range in age from six to twelve years old, and a great deal of time is spent coming and going, gathering up materials, or sitting and listening while the teacher tells one group or another what she expects. The teacher seems tired and impatient. My daughter never quite seems to understand what she is to do. Much later, I learn that this teacher has no Special Education training whatsoever. She is just another tired teacher, ready to retire, who has been given a small class full of "special" children to teach.

We're still doing the same amount of homework—and I start to believe that anything that Hilary is learning, she is learning at home with us. But at such a cost. Now not only are there tears, but raised voices, and arguments—and sometimes, refusal.

Later, much later, I learn that according to School Board policy, we should never have been required to do homework like this. In fact, homework is only permitted *after* Grade 3, and then for twenty minutes a night. Only then do I understand that, by complying all these years to each classroom teacher's homework demands, I have actually hidden my daughter's problems. That by destroying my home life with her, I have enabled the school to avoid acknowledging that Hilary was not learning. When I finally understand this, I feel anger at the way the school's burden so easily became my own. As well, I feel ashamed that I have been just the kind of mother my own mother was—a woman who sided with the school, a woman who tried to look like a team player, a woman who wanted to be understood as a "good mother."

*

The end of Grade Five. We receive a letter along with Hilary's last report card. Funding for the special Learning Disabilities class has dried up, and Hilary will attend Grade Six in a regular classroom. I meet with the school, and they assure me that this is a Good Thing. That Hilary will be happier integrated in the regular classroom, because, after all, a segregated setting is stigmatizing for these children.

Hilary's Learning Disabilities classroom teacher makes up little certificates with a picture of an eagle on the front, and a note inside telling the children that, now that they are no longer in the special class, they are ready to fly like the eagle.

As I read this note to my daughter, I recall how the school had assured me that the special class was just the right thing, and had dismissed my concerns about the stigmatizing effects of being segregated. I recall how I recently overheard the little girl down the street, who has been her friend for years, tell my daughter, "You know, I can be your friend on the weekends and at night, but I can't play with you at school, because it's not good for me. So don't try to play with me at school, okay?" I recall how the school assured me that the special classroom would enable Hilary to learn. I recall how I spend my evenings teaching her what she has not understood each day.

As I look at the card with the eagle on it, I recall all these things, taste the bile in my throat, hug my daughter and say "That's great, honey, you'll do really well in your new class next year." She's so pleased, and so proud, that it would feel mean-spirited of me to do anything else. Sometimes "whatever it takes" means you have be part of the lie.

*

Grade Six, and surprisingly, the regular classroom is going well. Hilary's teacher is very structured and stays every night after school to do homework with her. I cannot believe how much time we all have in the evenings, or how pleasant life can be when we are not fighting over schoolwork.

Still, I wonder how Hilary will manage next year in junior high school, when she has to move to eight different teachers a day in a school of seven hundred children, and when her social life is already filled with taunts and incredible sorrow. Will she be one who falls through the cracks? Will she be one who is driven to drugs or the wrong crowd because she feels she has no choice?

I meet with the vice principal and resource teacher at the junior-high Hilary will attend the next year to ask about their services. They provide me with a very short list. They also suggest I send my daughter to a two-week camp focusing on organizational skills, that I hire a tutor for Math and English from a private school for kids "like her," that I sign Hilary up for a computer keyboarding class, that I send her to a special summer camp for children with Learning Disabilities to help build up her self esteem.

The services they suggest are costly and involve additional work for Hilary over and above regular school. The responsibility has been clearly laid out. This is going to be our job, not the school's. As I walk out of this meeting, I feel surprisingly satisfied. I think I am finally beginning to understand what the rules are. It is a freeing realization.

I have always been a strong supporter of public education. I have always wanted Hilary to attend a community school that she can walk to, that her neighbors attend, and that we as parents contribute to. I have always believed in the principle of inclusion of *all* children in regular classrooms—I think the benefits for children who are "normal" are as great as they are for the children who are "different." However, beliefs can be challenged, and my daughter's future is at stake. And so, I start to enquire about private schools for children with Attentional and Learning Difficulties. Sometimes, "whatever it takes" means parking your principles and doing what needs to be done.

I am told we are too late to apply for next year. I apply anyway. I do this despite my husband's distinct lack of enthusiasm for placing his child in a "special school." I do this even though my daughter's current school warns me that this is a terrible mistake. I do this although we cannot possibly afford the tuition. I do this despite my own hopes of returning to school to complete a PhD in the fall. I do this, in short, on my own, with little confidence and few resources. I feel the fear, and I do it anyway.

I say, "Whatever it takes."

*

June. I receive a phone call from one of the private schools. A place is available, are we still interested?

My husband and I have talked about this. He's not so sure. Perhaps she'll be embarrassed to go to a school for kids with Learning Disabilities. Perhaps it won't make any difference anyway. Certainly, we cannot afford it.

My daughter and I have talked about this. She's pretty sure, then she's not. Maybe it won't work. Maybe it'll be lonely and stigmatizing, like the special class. Maybe it would be better to go to school with her friends—well, with the kids she knows.

I am weeping. I swallow hard and say, "Yes. Yes. We are still interested."

*

Epilogue

The year I said yes, the year I refused to play on the team any longer, was the year I began to get my daughter back. Despite my trepidation over what she might miss from not attending a community school, despite my misgivings about the legitimacy of her diagnosis, despite the worry that this would just be one more false alley along which to become further lost.

I remember the first parent-teacher meeting at that school like it was yesterday. The teacher sat across from us, eyes open, and told me "Hilary is not keeping up with her homework."

My heart sank. I thought, "Of course she isn't. She's given up. She's learned that she can't do it properly. She's learned that to ask for help results in tears and arguments. She's learned instead to tell us, 'No, I have no work to do tonight.'" I thought, "I know where this conversation is going—I've been here before."

But this time, the teacher didn't ask me about the problems at home, or suggest we have Hilary's medication levels checked, or ask me what I was going to do about it. Instead, she said, "So what I'm thinking is this. I'm thinking that you need to be taken off homework detail. I think this needs to belong to Hilary and me. I'm cutting you off."

It was a simple plan. Hilary either did her homework, or she stayed after school to catch up. And if she stayed after school, we were to devise some kind of "consequence" to compensate for the fact that we had to pick her up. The teacher facilitated these arrangements. *Facilitated* them.

It chagrins me to admit how hard it was for me to let the old homework routine go. I had to think long and hard about that one. Was my own sense of maternal worth so tied up in producing a good child and looking like a good mother that I was willing to torture all of us just to appease the school? Was I such a polite, compliant, middle-classed woman that the thought of truly resisting escaped me?

To be honest, I'm not sure. But I do know that letting go and letting the teacher own this problem was a terrible struggle for me. Not that I had loved our daily battles over homework or that I believed it was my job to teach Hilary. But for me, letting that homework go meant surrendering control, releasing my daughter to the world, and to herself. It was both exhilarating and terrifying.

It took almost a year, but—by God—she did it. With her teacher's guidance, she took responsibility for her own learning, in school and at home. And she has continued to do so ever since.

Six months later, she managed another thing I had never dared hope for. She became the best friend of someone in her classroom. I cannot tell you how much joy it gave me to pick up the phone and hear someone on the other end ask to speak with Hilary. Every night. Sometimes two or three times a night. It was wonderful.

I also have to admit how frightened I was for her—to see her open up to another child. I remained vigilant, holding my breath, listening for clues of cruelty from my daughter's end of the phone calls. I'm ashamed to admit that I let those suspicions color the way I treated my daughter's friend—I anticipated the scorpion's sting, and withheld both my trust and my gratitude. By way of excuse, all I can say is that watching Hilary endure all those hurts made me careful and—yes—smaller.

When Hilary began at the special school, I sought a Ritalin-free trial. I figured that now that she was in a "proper" school, she would no longer need to be medicated. The school, miraculously, was willing, and all of us—teacher, parent and child—monitored the situation to see whether good teaching in an appropriate educational setting might replace undesired medication.

Being either a very slow learner or an incurable skeptic, I have repeated this request each year since. Last year, after only a couple of days, Hilary put a stop to it, and said she needed the medication to help her concentrate.

Hilary continues to use her medication—as she always has—to help her with schoolwork only. She has never taken it on weekends or during vacations. There is still a part of me that feels uncomfortable with this—that worries that the medication is a crutch or that the demands of school are not a "natural" or reasonable part of life.

I suppose I believe that once she's finished with formal schooling she'll be able to let the medication go. However, I also realize that the choice will be hers and that, in the end, things are not turning out too badly for her, medication or not.

*

They say you should never look a gorilla in the eye—gorillas perceive a direct gaze as a challenge and will either attack or run away. Speaking with Hilary used to be like that. The only times we could talk were in the car or while watching television. Anything else was too threatening—she'd just shut down.

Since getting my daughter back—and I really do think of it that way—I know again how blue and clear her eyes are, how open her face, how kind and intelligent she is. Since Hilary came back, she looks me—and the world—in the eye, neither flinching nor fighting.

It's been a long trip, from that winter morning at the bus stop, through innumerable doctors, specialists, teachers, camps, workshops, and tutors, through tears, and rage, and—always—worry. But I think we're clear now. I think we're safe.

The F Word
Stacey Anderson

Friends,

People often ask politely, "soooo, what *is* wrong with Chase?"
"How *do you pay* for all those medical bills?" In the beginning, it was
actually entertaining to have the random (haven't heard from you in ten
years) phone calls, emails, and far-removed Facebook friends inquire
about my child's condition. I found it particularly odd that someone who
you barely know is sending a message with the preface, "I know it is
none of my business, but…" Exactly, it is none of your business! I never
was rude and always replied in a short and sweet manor. I was more
drawn to the friends or acquaintances who approached me with "I have
a similar situation, let me know if you need guidance" messages.

But, the thing that I remember most is the calls that I never got.
Yeah, Yeah. I know. It IS time to move on, and I have. But, I am sure
that many can relate—when dealt with a personal crisis, sometimes you
expect more from people. Sometimes, you didn't want the nosey
questions regarding the latest test or surgery, but rather the "how are
YOU doing?" or "do YOU need anything?" Not pity, not sympathy, just
genuine conversation. Then, a revelation! I was looking in the mirror at
the person who I should have been relying on the most.

I always joke that after the first year (the hardest) was past us and
Chase started sleeping, I was finally a flower that bloomed. I was
extremely sleep deprived. When I finally started to put things in
perspective, I reflected on the first year and appreciated the true
friendships that I made. I also learned to summarize his health in 25
words or less (best advice I ever got), because I don't have to explain his
personal issues. And, I left my venting or questions for my friends that
could relate and Facebook forums specific to his diagnosis(es).

My delivery with Chase was torture, no less. I remember it like
yesterday; whoever said that you forget it, was clearly not in my
delivery room! Not only did my body reach new heights in pain, I felt
like I could surpass anything. It truly gave me a level of internal
confidence. Just two weeks after his birth (when I knew something was
wrong), I found that I would need to reach back to that space, deep

inside my soul for courage and strength. It also taught me a valuable lesson; I can only depend on me. I am the captain of this ship, solo. I can't expect the unexpected from those who are a part of my world; I can only rely on my internal motivation. This is said not to discount the people closest to me that provided strength and encouragement during these times, but only to point out the internal transformation that takes place when a crisis enters your life. I truly think that my DNA changed, to put it a bit softer, probably I experienced an internal metamorphosis.

I would consider myself a "good" person *before*. I am honest to admit there was a slight misdirect in personal confidence, empowerment, and focus. I

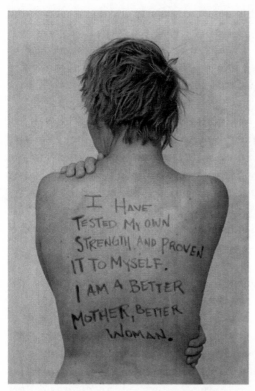

don't wish this journey on anyone, yet I wouldn't trade it for the world. I have tested my own strength and proven it to myself. I am a better mother, a better woman. I see the small things, appreciate the medium sized successes and embrace the large blessings.

In case you didn't notice, medical terms have not been mentioned. It is purely about the journey, most importantly, the selection. I have strong belief in faith and destiny. I was selected to be the mom of these boys, triumphs, tribulations, giggles, and puke. It's not perfect, and even today, I have prayed for more strength—juggling it all still proves challenging.

This morning was tough. While doing a tube feeding (don't ask what is in it), it exploded in my kitchen—at least 20 feet—at 8:00 a.m. (pre-coffee). I didn't get in the shower until 12:00 and didn't eat my soggy cereal until 12:30. I'm sure that I will be finding green slime in my hair two years from now. It wouldn't have been so bad, but it also happened yesterday, and the day before. I was tired, frustrated, and out of gas (mentally).

When I want to recharge, Erma Bombeck never fails to lift me up. She is my favorite author when I need that extra boost of, "come on Stace, you can do this!" She has a wonderful piece on what makes a mother special. It reminds us that we were chosen to guide our complex need children. Her focus is on love and patience and has a sprinkle of spiritual guidance. As parents, we must encourage each other not to ponder the sad times, rough nights, and the unknown future. But rather, we must realize that we were chosen for this journey because we are divine, we rise above pity, and we promote strength and independence. Bombeck claims that our children (just the way they are) are a precious gift; we were chosen, not by accident.

My favorite quote reads, "Yes, here is a woman whom I will bless with a child less than perfect. She doesn't realize it yet, but she is to be envied. She will never take for granted a 'spoken word.' She will never consider a 'step' ordinary. When her child says 'Momma' for the first time, she will be present at a miracle, and will know it" (Bombeck)! This sums it up: miracles now have new meaning to us. We know the true meaning of life and recognize the gift. Bombeck adds a veil of spirituality, saying, "I will permit her to see clearly, the things I see...ignorance, cruelty, prejudice...and allow her to rise above them. She will never be alone. I will be at her side every minute of every day of her life, because she is doing my work as surely as if she is here by my side." We should be proud of our strength; we are to be envied. At the end, Bombeck states (as God is describing the Special Needs mother), "'And what about her Patron saint?' asks the angel, his pen poised in mid-air. God smiles, 'A mirror will suffice.'" Here is to you, and your new-found strength!

Resource

Bombeck, Erma. "The Special Mother." *Our-Kids*. Our-Kids, 2012. Web. 20 Sept. 2013.

Thinking Lately
Amanda Apgar

I've been thinking a lot lately about hurt and love and friends, and alone-ness, and support, and being a parent of a kid who isn't like other kids. And grief. I have been thinking about grief.

Yesterday I felt like I had a bit of a breakthrough. My therapist, as it turns out, has a daughter who has Down syndrome, and knowing this has been really comforting for me, because I know she really, *really* understands what I am going through, and when she makes suggestions to me about how I might think about Jane and this time in our life, I trust her. This is different from how *most* people in my life have been able to listen and speak back to me. By no fault of their own, by nobody's doing, it just seems like it has been really hard to talk about Jane and my feelings about this, hard in the sense that my listeners just don't know how to deal. I don't know how to deal, and I don't expect anybody else to know how.

But, so, yesterday my therapist looked me in the eye and said, "It *is* possible for Jane to have a disability or a neurological impairment, and at the same time, for everything to be wonderful and okay."

I have been sort of talking about how I am waiting for things to be okay, for Jane to be okay, for the end of this delayed-ness and questioning and wondering. And how I think that if there is an end or an end in sight then maybe I can start to feel better and feel secure, and if there is going to be an end to this—a time when Jane is all caught up and doesn't have any underlying condition or impairment but is just like every other kid—then it is at this end that things will be wonderful and okay and we will have our little kid that we thought we would have.

My therapist, who has a kid who is developmentally delayed, looked me in the eye and said that these seemingly exclusive things—disabilities and okay-ness—are not mutually exclusive at all. Moreover, she said I don't need to wait, shouldn't wait, for that diagnosis that says "Jane has X and we will treat it in this way and she will/will not recover in X years," but that I might possibly be able to be right here and now aware that Jane isn't actually okay *right now* but that things are truly *okay*, and may be wonderful indeed.

And when my therapist told this to me and I knew she was telling me the truth from her life, I believed her. Last night, while I put Jane to sleep, and I lay down next to her and she gently played with my hair until she dozed off, I thought to myself, *If this is the best it is going to get, then that's totally okay.* And I meant it; I believe it. She is a wonderful and sweet person, and I love her and I feel fortunate to have such a nice baby, and I can maybe begin to deal better with the ways she is different from other babies.

I think this is an important step for me, though it does not come without it's own little bits of grief. Letting this in, this realization that this might be the best it is going to get, still comes with little pangs of sadness, of course. Okay-ness is okay-ness, not bliss. These incremental steps forward and back and even the standing still can be simultaneously hopeful and grief-stricken, and this is just a lot to manage. Which is why I think, sometimes, it is hard for people I love, for people who are close to me, to deal with it.

One of the very hardest things about this process has been trying to express my worry about Jane and her development, and being told that I was wrong to think those things or worry in that way, because Jane is just *fine*. There have been times in the past year when I felt that I had to try and *persuade* people close to me to see that Jane wasn't like other kids. *"She's her own person. She'll do it when she is ready!"* Other kids Jane's age usually chew food. *"Jane is wonderful!"* I know, I know Jane is *wonderful.* So painful. So hard. No judgment, and no blame. It's all hard. But, the last thing I really need is a lesson in how to manage my own unmanageable situation, and, honestly, least of all from someone who has no reference point for dealing with such a situation.

This, what I am describing, this super-positive response, I think comes from a desire to comfort me, and for that I am thankful and I DO get it, but nonetheless what this response does is completely foreclose on my attempts to express my worries and fears. The loving response that says, "What you are saying about Jane being different is irrelevant because you, and I, love Jane no matter what," effectively tells me that there is no space for me to express the thoughts that haunt my days. And, what I am describing is different from the optimistic cheerleading coming from so many friends and readers; "She'll catch up in no time!" and "She is doing so well and making so many improvements!" Thank you. There are improvements to be made, and I am comforted by the acknowledgement.

Other people I am close to have been so magnificent: listening and trying to understand without pretending to know. Sometimes, getting a text from a friend that read, "thought of you and Jane, cried with joy when I learned she stood up," or something like that, has made me feel like I was *the most loved* person on Earth. Some close friends have become less close and have perhaps allowed distance to mitigate the discomfort or confusion surrounding me, The Sad And Confused Friend With The At-Risk Kid. I find this easy to understand. How can we deal? How can I, we, deal with navigating this unpredictable territory—at once hopeful and full of dread? Peaceful, even happy at times, and angry, confused, depressed just as often? I have no answer, I do not judge, I only can say that some things have made me feel good and okay and that others that have caused me stress.

There is so much grief surrounding all of this. Little concessions that have to be made—*Okay, Jane is 17 months old and still doesn't say a single word*—and with each, there is a little lump in my throat. And how hard that must be for those around me... how can they know which milestone Jane failed to accomplish this month, the reason for my sullen mood. And why should I be at all frustrated by such an attempt to jolt me out of it with a bit of reasoning and tough love? I don't know. If this is the best that it is going to get, and if I can admit that this is lovely and wonderful, and Jane is wonderful and I love her, I find that I still easily slip into grief, and I have no reserve of grace.

A Rose by Any Other Name
Jennifer Meade

"You know," John said to me as we pulled into the parking lot of the Institute for Human Disability, a building as unattractive as its name suggests. "*Nothing* is going to change, no matter what she tells us today. He is still going to be our son."

That is so typical of my husband. Clarity. Integrity. He doesn't say much but what he does say is spot-on, which is more than I can say for myself. I *need* to talk, as though keeping my mouth moving is the emotional equivalent of treading water.

"You're right," I said haltingly, trying to mirror the conviction and confidence he had. But in all honesty, I didn't understand what he meant. I so desperately wanted to have his faith, my heart yearning to feel it in my blood and bones like he did. I'm his mother, for God's sake. What is wrong with me?

We walked through the doors and made our way to the doctor's makeshift office on the seventh floor.

"Excuse the mess," she said. "We're undergoing remodeling."

I can relate, I thought to myself. We sat down across from her at a long metal table, our bodies shifting in the stiff chairs while a stack of papers lay there mitigating the distance between the son we knew and the one we were about to meet.

Like any sensitive professional about to deliver bad news, she started with his strengths, deftly handling that with more sincerity than most had done before. The fact that she kept talking for so long caught me off guard, but despite her best efforts, I couldn't help but wonder when the axe was going to fall. I had heard this talk before, in different ways, from different people whose job it was to guide parents like us through the unfamiliar terrain of having a *special* child.

But the axe never quite fell as hard as I had come to expect since the days I had first noticed my son was different. The doctor said so many things in the time we sat at that cold metal table, but six of her words bore down deep into my soul, grabbing me by the collar and shaking me, hard. These six words were ones I never expected to hear. In my son's short life, we had gone through so many evaluations to try and make sense of our lives and the inner workings of his mind, from the time he was a baby until now, and we'd always ended up with more questions than answers. And now, as he neared two and a half, came six small and ordinary words that held the power to stir my soul.

"You'd better start saving for college."

I don't remember much else from what she said that day, save for a few well-timed nods and murmurs of assent. The rest just washed over me in waves, sucking me into an undertow of good news I never anticipated. I knew I should feel thrilled, but her words came as such a shock that I couldn't get my bearings. In just a few seconds, I found myself in a tortured struggle, hating myself for not feeling purely ecstatic, yet feeling overwhelmed by a nervous and conditional joy. Maybe this sounds peculiar. It's just that in the past two years I had become very good at one thing—worrying about my son—and with that, figuring out the next steps I needed to take to get him help. And now with six small words, she forced me to look beyond the next step, beyond even the next day. The act of self-preservation had taught me not to think that far.

In the daily experience of living with a child with whom you cannot communicate, who challenges your every instinct about how to mother, it's hard to indulge in thinking about the future. You're much too busy figuring out how to get through the day. But now in the span of a few seconds, with six words other parents would have found trivial, the doctor had thrust me into this new and unexpected sea of possibilities I had not yet had the room to consider. Her explanations and prognostications sloshed around me in unrelenting waves as she continued speaking, and I struggled to find something I could grasp onto to make sense of it all. Living life preparing for the worst had left me utterly unprepared for the possibility of hope.

My neurons competed in vain to mine the datafield of information she had dropped in our laps. My body felt rocked by waves, and my eyes kept searching for the shore. But as I treaded water, I began to slowly comprehend my husband's words. Her lengthy and careful evaluation did not take away the son I knew. I just still couldn't tell what it *gave* me. All I knew for certain was that I would go home that day to a life that was the same, and a boy who was the same, just with new words to describe the world we lived in every day.

Could this time we spent with her bring closure to this seemingly endless journey to name this? All these months of angst-filled searching to label what "this" was, what our son had, thinking that a single word could make sense of our daily realities and somehow tell us how to live. And here she had given that to us, wrapped in a careful package of observations and recommendations and tied with a neat diagnostic bow. Yet now that I could hold it in my hands and speak it on my tongue, it held no power. It was neither beginning nor end, neither the gift nor curse I had expected, yet feared. I felt like Dorothy arriving in Oz, forced to confront the impotence of all that she had put her faith in.

The doctor began to finish up her monologue. As she talked, my mind started to wander, transporting me back to a trip I took to Italy as a teenager. I can picture it like it was yesterday, sitting in the piazza soaking up the sun, drinking in the energy of so many beautiful people who *are* beautiful simply because they *think* they are beautiful. They have something to say because they think they have something to say, enough to fill up three hours' time in the same café, philosophizing in a romantic dance of gesture and sound.

The doctor coughed. Perhaps she could sense I was no longer there, and I was jolted back to reality as quickly as I left it. That world seemed so glamorous and so far from mine, not because I wouldn't savor the chance to sip cappuccino and watch the pigeons swoop and swoon over crumbs of biscotti, but because the thought of taking three hours for myself seemed so luxurious, it almost felt criminal.

Perhaps that is what fills my heart feel with such heaviness that I can barely breathe sometimes. Nothing really changes now that this rose has a name. Our son is still our son, the same shimmering blue eyes, the same endless ball of energy he was the day before we came home with that stack of papers so high that I still can't bring myself to crack their pages. The thought of it alone gives me a mental paper cut. No matter what we call this, it doesn't make the *sturm und drang* of our daily lives any easier, more manageable or any different at all. It just adds more layers of complexity to our already complicated, stretched-thin, stressed-out lives. Only now we have a tidy diagnostic code we can put after it for emphasis.

So there is no going back to Italy right now, save for in my head. Because what did change with this diagnosis is that it showed me *which* mountain range I'm climbing. Before this, I was climbing blind, no map or headlamp to guide me. I am still climbing. But when I have time to pick up my head and take a breath, I can pause, breathe deep, and survey the scene around me. I can take in the color and the texture of the landscape. I can now see other climbers, ahead of and behind me, and maybe every now and then catch up with one to swap stories about which rock to scrabble to next and where to take shelter when the winds whip through the crevasse at night.

Eventually, I know that I will come to see the mountains for all the rugged, imperfect, irreplaceable beauty they possess. But for now the scrabbling is the next best task before me. Because everything and nothing changes now that we have a name for whatever *this* is. My bright-eyed son wakes up each day and in the complicated calculus of the day and this "disorder" and whatever kind of sleep we've all had and how much we've got to do that afternoon and the phone calls that must be returned and the mental breakdowns and the hopes and the extinguished hopes competing desperately for center stage, life does go on.

We keep on scrabbling. He keeps on learning and so do we sometimes, despite our best efforts. Our boys make us laugh. They make us cry, and we, the same for them. Our bills get paid, our dishwasher loaded, our laundry washed. There is no Special Needs Fairy Godmother who swoops down from above to take on the little tasks so we can tackle the big ones. We just bite off a little chunk of What Needs To Get Done and hope we don't choke this time.

Years have now passed since we sat at that table, the distasteful image of the Institute having long since receded in the rearview mirror of my mind, but memories of that day stay with me like muscle memory stays in my body. I know now that I did come home with a gift that day, just not the gift I had expected. I went there desperate for a name to make sense of the world I lived in, and with that name, a healing balm to somehow soothe the pain of my failures as a mother to connect with my own child. I got that name, but in the end it gave me nothing. The real gift the doctor gave me was hope. And that hope was what transformed me.

I've come to understand now how little a name truly matters. Yes, it can put you on a path to getting more help for your child, and that is undoubtedly important. But the name in and of itself does not change your life. Nor does it tell you *anything* about who your child is or who he will become. And that name wields a frightening power. It makes it far too easy for the world outside to put my child in a box and that terrifies me. Many will choose to attach to the name and not to the boy behind it. And I shudder knowing that I may have to shield him from this for the rest of my life.

It all makes such visceral sense to me now, what my husband meant that day as we pulled into the parking lot full of nervous anticipation. Our precious son is still our son, and by whatever name, he smells as sweet. That was the lesson I needed to learn on my journey to mother a child with special needs. And through the transformative gift of hope, to come to believe in my blood and in my bones that my son will continue to grow, that his bud will open and reveal a beauty so extraordinary that its power will transform our lives. Indeed, he already has.

Challenges: Sometimes It Sucks
Mary E. Overfield

"You can't control the wind, but you can adjust your sails."
— Yiddish proverb

Growing up in a family who enjoyed sailing, I had always held this quote as one of my favorites. Back in high school, when I had first heard it, I could easily relate the words to a good day of sailing; high winds or no winds, the sails could be adjusted to make the most of the wind that was available. After college, I got married, and we had our first daughter in October of 1995. Overall, "life was good," as the saying goes. Life had not thrown many curve balls my way until the birth of our daughter, Megan. Although my pregnancy had been relatively uneventful and Megan was born during a routine scheduled C-section, her birth was anything but routine. Life as we knew it for my husband, twenty-one month old daughter, and me, was forever changed on a July afternoon in 1997. As Megan was immediately whisked away to special care nursery to access her low Apgar scores, I recall feeling as if I was drowning in a sense of overwhelming dread. It was as if someone had sucked the wind out of my sails. The birth of a child is supposed to be a happy, joyful occasion. How could I feel so helpless? What was happening?

My husband came back to the delivery area with the doctor a short time later to report that one of Megan's lungs had collapsed and she was being transferred to another hospital to receive care in their NICU. My husband followed Megan to the hospital. As I laid there in my bed, post-surgery, still tied to an IV pole, feeling more scared and alone than I could ever recall feeling, the reality of the situation began to sink in. I realized then and there that I had absolutely no control over the situation at hand. And it sucked.

In the weeks and months to come, Megan eventually came home from the NICU on supplemental oxygen, along with a host of medical issues. As we began to navigate the unfamiliar waters of caring for a medically frail child, I remember thinking, how were other people continuing to sail easily through daily life while we were stuck dead in the water, with no prospect of wind for our sails? We were suddenly very isolated from the life we were living prior to Megan's birth. Friends did not know how to approach our situation, so they no longer called or visited. I guess it was easier to avoid than support. Our extended families struggled as well. All of our relatives lived out of town, and Megan became a "burden" who was keeping us from travelling, visiting, and participating in any family or recreational event that was not planned weeks or months in advance.

We tried our best to settle into a routine of medical appointments, therapy sessions, and frequent trips to the hospital and pharmacy. As I was sitting with Megan one morning in a hospital clinic waiting room, there was a beautiful painting of a sailboat on the wall. I remember looking at it with more than a slight sense of resentment, thinking I would most likely not be sailing much in this "new life" with Megan, and I already missed it. And suddenly, out of nowhere, that long-forgotten quote came to my mind. "You can't control the wind, but you can adjust your sails." I was keenly aware that I had no control over the fact that Megan was born with multiple disabilities, and she was not the same child we had envisioned for nine months. But maybe I could alter my sails a bit and learn to accommodate this new life better with some adjusting.

For the first three years of Megan's life, we seemed to be adjusting our sails every few months or so. There was the oxygen, then the seizure disorder, then the feeding tube, then the wheelchair—it seemed that every time we adjusted our sails to accommodate a new medical support, the wind would start blowing from a new direction. It was not until Megan was about five years old that I really began to settle into a familiar routine with her care. The winds were relatively steady, and our sails were adequately adjusted to accommodate them. Although I was feeling more confident about my role as mother to a special needs daughter, I was also feeling the eternity of the situation. And it sucked.

Other mothers were living through the typical stages of growth with their children, from feedings, to teething, to learning to walk, to starting preschool, and all the while, the common denominator was that each stage was temporary and led to new growth and skills for the children. Megan was in, and continues to be in, a permanent newborn stage, requiring around-the-clock care, a continuous feeding schedule, close supervision for safety and seizure precautions, and frequent diaper changes. Megan is completely dependent upon others for every single aspect of her care, and she is non-verbal and non-ambulatory, functioning at the level of a six-month-old baby. We have missed many family events due to the constraints of Megan's care, and we are not able to live spontaneously since everything we do now requires a great deal of long-term planning to accommodate Megan's care. There are no temporary stages for Megan, and she will most likely not gain any new skills. There is also the feeling of guilt that comes with the stress of caring for a sick child while the uncertainty of her life expectancy looms incessantly in the back of my mind. And that sucks.

It has been almost sixteen years since Megan was born, and over the years, I have learned that although I have no control over the winds of life, controlling my sails has helped me determine my direction, and at times, my speed in life. Megan has taught all of us to slow down and make the most of the scenery along the journey. Megan is almost always happy and finds the simplest things in life to be funny. She has a weak body, but a strong spirit, and in her own way, I believe she has adapted her spirit to make up for the lack of control over her body. I am quite certain that Megan is responsible for the kind heart and giving soul of our older daughter. Although it is not the life journey we would have chosen, we have all changed for the better, discovering inner strength and heartfelt compassion that we may not have experienced without Megan in our lives. And that doesn't suck.

There are still days when I feel resentful, isolated, and overwhelmed. But then I try adjusting my sails to gain a different perspective. I have come to realize, most likely thanks to Megan, that I cannot control what happens *to* me, but I can control what happens *in* me. My quality of life is determined by the choices that I make, or how I adjust my sails. I can choose to be bitter and float aimlessly, or I can choose to be accepting of the wind in my life and adjust to it the best that I can. I choose the latter.

Kin

Sally Bittner Bonn

I couldn't take my eyes off you. I recognized myself in the cut of your jaw, not because our faces have the same shape but because of the energy, the intent. You had that look about you that I sometimes wear. That look that says you know there may be many eyes in the room watching you. Watching you do what you always do, whether in a room full of people, or just the two of you.

I saw the two of you come in, during the opening band, a few rows in front of where David and I were sitting, where an aisle cuts the front of the orchestra section in half from front to back. I saw the three small green lights on his power chair glide into place. I saw you with your gentle confidence and your graceful blonde hair. Even in the dark, I saw the vibrant youth in both of you. I nudged David, nodded in your direction. Silently we delighted in the comfort of having a young man in a power chair in the room, sharing this musical experience with us.

During the intermission you set to work removing his jacket. You held his body with the familiarity of someone who has done this many times. You shifted his weight, supported his shoulder to keep him from toppling. I was surprised. From the back he looked so stable, strong, square-shouldered. But then I noticed the lateral supports on the side of his chair. The small rectangles that extend out to support his ribs on either side. Oscar, too, needs lateral supports to keep him from tipping. A year or so earlier and I wouldn't have had any idea what lateral supports were or how to identify them on a wheelchair.

Your nimble fingers unzipped the orange backpack, hanging from the hook on the back of your fella's wheels. Maybe to retrieve his phone or return his wallet. Maybe he bought a limited edition poster on the way in. We did.

David and I asked each other again and again, "What should we do?" "Should we go say hi?" "What do we say?" I wanted to talk to you. I wanted to make the connection. I wanted both of you to know our son would soon be getting a power chair. I wanted you to know you had kin in the room. I wanted to acknowledge our kin in the room.

You see, this was the first time I'd been away from my boy overnight. Eleven days before our son's third birthday, David and I drove the seven hours to Ann Arbor to hear the Fleet Foxes in concert.

We enjoyed seven hours of uninterrupted adult conversation in the car. Here we felt free and also vulnerable.

It had been twenty-two months, since we found out that Oscar would need a power chair. We were now excited about the mobility he would soon experience and also still getting used to the idea. I didn't have the reference point at the time to discuss brands with the two of you, "Oh we're looking at a Permobil for our son, do you like yours?" Or features, "We noticed you have one of those sit-to-stand wheelchairs. We wonder if Oscar will get one of those someday!"

But, I chickened out. We stayed in out seats. Robin Pecknold's honied voice came sweeping out over all our heads. You settled your arm around your guy, leaned your head into his shoulder. I reached over and rested my hand on David's corduroyed knee. I didn't yet know how to broach this kind of conversation. I didn't yet know if it's okay to single someone out because of a wheelchair. And perhaps the two of you would like to be left on your own to enjoy your date, to be out in public and not have the wheelchair be a central point of focus. Besides, perhaps I'd come across as too excited, too awkward, too obvious.

Nonetheless, that night you carried my hope far into the future. Hope that my son may find a mate as loyal and smart and steadfast as you, or at least as you appeared to be from our vantage point. Hope that his days will be numbered high enough to attend colossal music events with someone, other than his parents, who loves him fiercely and gently.

In you, I saw a normalcy I could not see before.

116

Viable Faith
Tracey Trousdell

My husband Jordan and I walk in silence; no words exist to comfort us. We keep a safe distance apart as we cross the slippery parking lot. Somehow we know that if we touch, we will both fall to pieces.

A few minutes prior, we were sitting amongst the other couples in the ultrasound waiting room, excited to put a picture to the baby we had been getting to know over the past nineteen weeks. We were already well-versed in the crackled "whoosh" of its heart rate through the doppler, and I was becoming accustomed to the fluttering in my belly that had recently turned into full-fledged kicks.

We watched the clock, anxious to be called in for the exam. We held hands and recounted the thrill of the first images of our older daughter Rio, almost exactly three years prior. We whispered jokes and took silly pictures of our shoes in an effort to pass the time. They are the last memento I have of "before."

Now walking from the clinic my legs buckle beneath me, as if a sign that my world really is collapsing. The weight these legs have been carrying for thirty-three years is suddenly too much to bear. I grab the car door to support me, and as I slide in to my cold seat my body numbs to match my emotions. I try to make sense of what we've just learned but it is impossible. There are no explanations. I have a hard time believing this is not a nightmare that I will soon wake up from.

"Not viable."

A million thoughts swirl around in my head, but all that matters is that our baby is going to die.

No kidneys. How is that even possible? Every part of her is perfect with the exception of one fatal flaw. I had done everything right—how could something so wrong be happening?

I beg for them to be mistaken. I pray to God or someone—*anyone who is listening*—to save my baby. Whatever complications come along with her, I'm prepared to handle.

Please, just let my daughter live.

But my pleading doesn't help. Although my heart knows her intimately, I never meet my baby. My body is confused, not realizing there is no baby to bond with or provide for. Later I cling to her tiny, tear-stained footprints and heart-shaped box of ashes as the only physical evidence I have of her existence. Physically and mentally, I am broken.

Or so I believe.

After much grieving and desperately looking for answers, I begin to accept that I was meant to lose her and have my strength challenged. This baby girl who never drew breath prepared me for future challenges I had no idea were coming. Her loss gave me the reassurance that I would love a baby no matter what, and she showed me that I am stronger and more resilient than I knew possible.

I used to despise hearing, "You're never given more than you can handle." Of course I always thought it was those who hadn't faced any adversity who were the first to spout off such clichés. Now, however, after facing adversity myself, I may be starting to believe there is some truth to it.

*

Ten months later, I'm on my back staring at the coved plaster ceiling and four blue walls that seem to be closing in around me. I am allowed to get up to use the bathroom, but must remain lying flat at all other times. I'm bored and often lose track of entire portions of the day, but at least I have everything I need at arm's reach. My resourceful husband has built me a table level with our bed, so I can access everything without sitting up. I have water, remote controls, vitamins, medications, hand sanitizer, ChapStick, my cell phone, books, magazines, movies, a laptop, and my iPod. There're extra blankets, a photo collage of Jordan and Rio, and even a small fridge stocked with food and dishes beside the bed. To say I'm taken care of is an understatement. My support circle of friends and family has rallied; I'm seldom left alone.

I'm twenty-four weeks pregnant and confined to complete bed rest at home. Although we survived the nineteen-week ultrasound without any devastating news like last time, other complications have arisen threatening early delivery. I am teetering precariously on the brink of viability for any pregnancy, but things are even more complicated by the fact that I'm carrying identical twins.

Doctors have given me no reason to believe I can't carry the babies close to term if I remain in bed. Although scared, I feel blessed and hopeful, believing we've been given twins as a way of somehow compensating for our previous loss. I follow doctor's orders to the letter and am confident that my babies will make it. Once again however, I am reminded that some things happened beyond my best intentions and are out of my hands. I awake one night in terror: I'm having contractions and I'm only twenty-six weeks pregnant.

Twelve hours after I'm admitted to hospital, I give birth by emergency C-section while under general anaesthetic. Jordan is not allowed in the operating room and only sees our babies whisked by on their way to the neonatal intensive care unit. Several hours later, I am wheeled into the NICU on a stretcher to meet them. They are covered in tubes and wires with machines breathing for them. We are not allowed to touch them. They are unbelievably small, but I am more fascinated by the sheen and transparency of their skin that shouldn't have seen the light of day for more than three months. I am in disbelief that these children, so foreign looking to me, need me to have a mother's strength when I am at my weakest. Our baby boys, Asher and Nolan, weigh a scant two pounds each and are in a fight for their lives.

The boys make it through the first twenty-four hours, then forty-eight. At the seventy-two hour mark, I exhale for the first time, but our relief is short lived. On their fourth day of life, we find out that Asher has had a massive brain hemorrhage. He will live, but with what quality we don't know. We are devastated and fear the future, but are forced to remain in the present. The boys have a long, hard journey ahead of them in the NICU, and keeping them alive day-by-day has to be our focus.

Given no other choice, we develop a routine for this life we have been thrown into: pumping breast milk, visiting the boys, calling up between visits, and trying to keep life at home as normal as possible for Rio. Somehow Jordan even manages to go to work, and often I am jealous for his short escape from our new reality.

Our visits to the hospital are predictable. We meet with doctors to discuss plans and treatments. We review progress and concerns with our nurses. We watch cardiac monitors plummet, then level out, then plummet again. We give the boys skin to skin contact when they are stable, and we stare at them through their plastic incubators when they are not. We analyze weights and feeds down to the gram. We see their skin turn a startling bluish-grey just as quickly as we see it return to pink. We cry, and sometimes in spite of ourselves, we laugh. After what seems like an eternity, we bring our boys home together after one hundred fifty-two days in the hospital.

We aren't naive; we know that a birth as early as Asher and Nolan's, with the many serious complications it included, means they will likely not walk away unscathed. Although worry about the boys is ever present and sometimes crippling, we enjoy finally being together as a family.

*

The doctor, and her office, are unfamiliar to me. I have been to this building several times for other appointments in the past year since the boys have been home from the hospital, but had no idea this hallway of offices even existed, nor had I heard of the medical specialty "physiatry" until we were referred to her. Jordan and I sit nervously with the boys on our laps, making idle chit chat with our physio-therapist who is there to support us. Rio, now an energetic almost-five year old, cannot sit still, disinterested in the meagre collection of toys available to her.

The doctor comes in to greet us. She is somewhere around my age, which always makes me feel a little bit inadequate. She is friendly and tells us she too is a mom of twins, not much older than ours. We talk a bit about the boys' history as she reviews Asher's chart, and she is pleased to know how healthy they have been since they were discharged. We give her highlights of the boys' development, but it's difficult to finish a sentence because they are babbling loudly and Rio is demanding our attention.

As the doctor examines Asher, she asks a lot of questions and makes many observations. She compliments him often, telling him how bright and clever he is. When she finishes the exam she hands Asher back to me and sits down across from us.

"So Asher has Cerebral Palsy," she says slowly, but without hesitation. "Do you understand what that means?"

Jordan and I nod, as my eyes pool with tears. He squeezes my hand.

She gives us an empathetic smile then takes a deep breath and continues discussing type, severity, and prognosis, in as much detail as she can provide given how young he is. As she talks, I nod some more and say "mmm hmm" at the appropriate places, but I'm not really listening.

120

My thoughts trail off to the last sixteen months since Asher's brain hemorrhage. I spent hours reading on the Internet and making online friends with moms whose kids had CP. As much hope as I had, I was also a realist. I spent every waking minute with him, and he had an older sister and an identical twin to compare to; I knew that all of the delayed milestones could not be explained away by the prematurity. In the time since his bleed had been discovered, I had been preparing for this day. For every hour I spent researching, my heart breaking a little bit more with every click of the mouse, I doubled it grieving. Sometimes I told Jordan about my worries, but most of the time I kept them to myself. The looming diagnosis of CP was eating me up inside. So today, upon receiving the diagnosis, it's almost a relief.

The doctor grabs my attention fully again when she says that although she cannot be sure of what he will be capable of physically, she believes Asher is cognitively typical, and she has great expectations for his quality of life. Once again I'm able to exhale, if just for a moment. We quietly gather up the kids and walk out of the room, into our new world. Dreams for our future have not been shattered completely, but they will need to be re-adjusted.

*

At eighteen-month checkups with three separate doctors, we are assured that while he's late to walk, there is nothing of great concern. He's been late at sitting and crawling too, and those are now completely normal. I try not to worry.

Two years old now, and he's still not walking. He finally pulls himself up to furniture and can take a few steps holding someone's hands, but otherwise he's off balance and falls repeatedly.

A few more months, and we're back in that same office with the same doctor who has now become familiar to us.

"How's Asher been doing?" she asks.

"Great," we tell her, as Asher flashes her a bright smile and then continues to chat to Nolan who is playing with dump trucks in the far corner of the office.

She comments on how big the boys are getting and then the room falls silent because we can't deny why we're here any longer.

"Hi Nolan," she begins carefully, knowing by now how shy he is. She asks him if she can lie him on the table, and he tentatively agrees.

She then examines him with the same level of detail as she did Asher for the first time more than a year ago.

Then, as if déjà vu, she sits in the same chair and with the boys now back in our laps, we have a similar conversation. Although I'm not completely shocked, this time I listen to her more intently. I'd like to know how on earth Nolan has Cerebral Palsy too.

A year ago, if you'd told me Nolan would be diagnosed with CP, I would have laughed you out of the room—partly because I didn't think it was possible with no brain injury detected, but more importantly because I didn't believe our family could handle anything else. But over the previous months, I started to accept that Nolan's inability to walk steadily couldn't be explained away any longer. While I hoped and prayed that I was wrong, I knew in my heart a CP diagnosis was likely imminent.

Devastating? Yes. But unlike with Asher's diagnosis, this time I only had a few days of grieving and hating the world. We were becoming dangerously accustomed to receiving bad news, and somehow bouncing back from it was becoming surprisingly easier.

*

The tears usually come in the shower, driving with the rear view mirror tilted so the kids can't see my reflection, or in bed at night when Jordan is already asleep. Positive as I try to be most of the time, I have my bad days. During the really tough times, I don't have the energy to hide it. I cry for what we have been through and even more for the uncertainty of the boys' future. Sometimes I don't think I can face any more, the stress tightening its grip and squeezing the breath out of me. Yet somehow I manage to get through one day, and then another, finally arriving back at a place of near—if not yet complete—acceptance. What other choice do I have? My children need me.

I have been tested enough. I have lost a child. I have delivered two more far too early. I have lived through months of uncertainty while my sons were hospitalized. I had not one, but two children diagnosed with Cerebral Palsy. On top of everything we've been through with the kids, I recently faced thyroid cancer—particularly distressing after watching my mom slowly die from breast cancer when I was a teenager.

That list of challenges is, on the one hand, a cry for justice, "Please stop, we've been through enough." But on the other hand, it's me yelling loud and proud, "Look what I've survived." It gives me faith that, like my boys, I am a fighter and can face my obstacles head on.

A friend going through hard times of her own recently asked me what I thought came first: my strength or the circumstances that forced me to find it.

I guess I'll never know. But does it matter? The important part is that somehow, the strength is there.

Splinter Skills
Jamie Pacton

When I think about my hopes for my son's future, I don't think college, kids, or Fortune 500 companies. Marriage, vacations, 401K's—these don't enter my head. I don't see him backpacking across Europe, sneaking out of the house, or visiting me in a nursing home.

For now, I just think about T-shirts. Rows and rows and rows of colorful, neatly folded T-shirts.

This is because a friend recently told me about an autistic adult she knows who loves folding laundry. When he was a kid, he relished folding all the laundry at home, so his wise mother promptly made that his job. Now, at twenty-two, he's successfully translated this passion to real employment. He takes the bus every day to a store in suburban Milwaukee where he folds and straightens endless piles of T-shirts for eight hours every day.

Is it fair, however, to call this a passion? Can one really be all that jazzed about folding laundry?

If you say no, then you've never parented an autistic child in the throes of an obsession. Kids on the spectrum stumble into the oddest, most eccentric corners of life. The lucky ones can easily translate their interests (the clinical term here is "splinter skills") into real-world employment. For those kids who find themselves needing to memorize the names of all the stars in the sky, or tinker endlessly with electronics, or forge steel in their garage with basic chemistry sets, there are jobs waiting for them as eccentric, brilliant, singularly-focused astronomers, engineers, and chemists. Others love less academic things that can still be translated to gainful employment—rare books, subway schedules, antique refrigerators, cattle chutes, and hundreds of other pursuits.

But, what about the other "other" kids—the ones like my sweet, severely autistic five-year-old, Liam? Unlike many of his autistic peers, he's not exhibited any clear splinter skills beyond a love of peanut butter and jelly and a surprising deftness with climbing the cabinets to steal hidden pieces of gluten-free gum. What if he never develops any of the "genius" aspects of autism and just ends up finding fulfillment in a simple, repetitive task like folding T-shirts? If that's enough for him, will that be enough for me?

I have to look this question straight on and really let it punch me a few times before I can think clearly here.

I mean, what about all those plans I had for play dates, the vacations we'd take together, and all the things he'd do that I didn't get around to doing? What about all those little ways that he was going to be because I wanted him to be that way?

Here's autism parenting lesson #1: things are not as you expected. Deal with it. Love the child you have, not the one you thought you earned/deserved/expected.

I know that sounds brutal—and it is at first—but there's a whole lot of good within this lesson. As a parent to a child with autism, I haven't given up on my son. I haven't lowered my expectations *tout court*. Rather, I've done what every parent gets around to doing eventually—usually after a decimating series of teenage years and the eventual reconciliation that follows everyone growing up a bit, children moving out and moving on, and the cycle of parenting beginning again—I've looked at my son for exactly who he is and removed all my expectations for who he should be from the equation.

Does this make me a better parent?

Of course not.

Do I feel smugly superior?

Oh no, and I often wish that I could still project my hopes, dreams, and expectations onto Liam.

But, the simple fact of the matter is that all of them slide off him like a runny egg on a mound of hash browns. He is fully his own being, and his autism ensures that he will not be the straight-A, soccer-playing, punk-rock-loving, free-thinking, surfer dude that I imagined I'd raise.

So, what kind of mom looks at her kid and thinks, "man, I hope you land a sweet gig folding T-shirts when you're in your early 20's?"

An autism mom, that's who.

The autistic man my friend told me about is happy. He has meaningful work, and he is respected for what he does. Any parent of a child with special needs could only dare to dream of so much.

Facing the future is a tough job. Looking ahead to the time when "everything that will be, already is," as Temple Grandin's mother puts it, terrifies me. But, if Liam can find something that he loves—whether it evolves into a splinter skill or not— then I think I can live with that.

After all, this is his life and his future we're talking about here, not mine.

I Was a Knucklehead

Heather Kirn Lanier

Lately, a story from my past has been replaying in my mind, one that makes me cringe at my former self. I once spent a summer working with a woman who was about four or five months pregnant. Each week, I watched her bump get just a bit rounder, until finally the summer ended, and she was not yet beach-ball bursting, and we parted ways. This was back when I was in my twenties, when motherhood for me was a foreign country I planned to enter someday but was otherwise happy to nod at from a distance.

About six months later, a friend asked if I'd heard about my former coworker's baby. I hadn't heard anything. I assumed the baby was out and about in the world and doing whatever it was that babies did. What *did* babies do? I didn't know. I was a busy grad student.

My friend said, "The baby has Down syndrome."

And my reply was, "Oh, how sad."

And that is the part that makes me cringe.

The friend agreed, it was sad. And then we talked about how sad it seemed. Down syndrome. It seemed like an end. Like a deflation. Like the helium party balloons all getting popped. We talked about how heartbroken she must have felt. We talked about how she would probably not want any other kids after that, since obviously she made Down syndrome babies, which, in my idiot mind, was a tragedy.

Again, I was a knucklehead.

The question I ask myself now is, why? Why did I think Down syndrome was such a warrant for grief? A few months later, I actually did see my former coworker from a distance. It was a far enough distance that it would have been awkward to shout hello. So I just went my way. But there's another reason I didn't rush up and say hi: I thought she was probably living in a shroud of grief. I imagined a black veil over her head. How sad, I still thought. All those months of pregnancy, of expectation and hope, and now she's caring for a Down syndrome baby. She must be miserable.

Good God, how I cringe at myself now.

Here is what I should have done. I should have jumped for joy at the birth of her child. I should have greeted her in the hall with a warm smile and a "Congratulations!" I might have asked how she was feeling, knowing what I now know about post-birth recovery and perineal tears and what-not. If she showed me pictures, I should have commented on how gorgeous her baby was. Because no doubt he probably was. And, because I now know a little about the risks that Down syndrome brings, I might have asked with compassion how his echocardiogram went, and if they liked their cardiologist at the children's hospital. And how was nursing?

But I say this all because I now live in the country of not only parenting but special needs parenting, because I now know what "echocardiogram" is, what "perineal tear" is, because I know how important it is to like your child's specialists, and I know how much of oneself one must give in order to get a child to latch late into the night.

Instead, I clammed up, believing she wouldn't want to talk about what in my mind was like birthing a funeral.

Again, I ask myself, why? Why did I ever think a child with Down syndrome was a bundle of grief, not joy? Because I thought a life of cognitive disability wasn't worth living? Or was less worthy of living? Was I really that ableist?

It's tough to admit, but yes, before Fiona I think I was probably ableist. Which means subconsciously I believed that an able-bodied life, in particular a *cognitively* able-bodied life, was superior to a disabled one.

Apparently others believed the same. In several regional studies, 80 to 90% of mothers chose to terminate their pregnancies when they learned through prenatal testing that their child had Down syndrome. Regional studies have their limitations, since they don't represent the full spectrum of a nation, and even before Fiona, I'd decided I could never terminate a wanted pregnancy simply because the baby wasn't chromosomally typical, but still, I think we can agree that there's a cultural bias against having a Down syndrome baby, or any baby, for that matter, with a chromosomal anomaly or special need. A baby that's not medically "perfect."

And for all the practical reasons, I get why. Fiona has an incredibly rare genetic deletion on the short arm of her fourth chromosome. Sometimes when I sneak a peek at the computer screen over the shoulder of one of Fiona's many specialists, my stomach sinks at the list of diagnoses. Atrial Septum Defect. Pulmonary Valve Stenosis. Hydronephrosis. Hypotonia. Febrile Seizures. Delayed speech. Delayed motor skills. The list goes one. It's a tall column of medical "problems." It seems like the older she gets, the more they add to that list. From a medical standpoint, she is far from "perfect."

But her life is not a bundle of grief. If you've met her, you know that Fiona adores being in this world. Really adores it! She is constantly clapping. She's smiling at least 50% of the time. My sister recently asked if, like a dolphin, Fiona's face just gave off the permanent impression of happiness. "No," I said. "She's that happy."

She seeks out strangers by eyeing them, cocking her head, and smiling, simply because she wants to connect. Just yesterday, a woman with dark-brimmed glasses and dangle earrings became enchanted with Fi at the grocery store. "Well, hello!" I heard someone say as I was scrutinizing the protein bar section. I turned around to see the woman at my cart, peering down at Fiona, like they were related.

"She's so friendly!"

I agreed.

"How old is she?"

"Sixteen months," I said. But of course Fiona looks five months. So I explained that I thought that was why people were often so captivated by her. Socially she's more advanced than she looks.

God bless this woman, who corrected my tendency toward uber-practical rationalizing. "Or it's her big soul!" she said.

"Well, yes," I said and laughed. "There's that too."

My girl's got a big soul. They haven't developed prenatal genetic testing for that yet.

Here's a helpful quote from *Wikipedia* of all places: "The ableist worldview holds that disability is an error, a mistake, or a failing, rather than a simple consequence of human diversity, akin to race, ethnicity, sexual orientation or gender." Sometimes I like to imagine that we flip the ableist worldview on its head. The condition Fiona has is extremely rare. 1 in 50,000. Sometimes I like to imagine a world where Wolf-Hirschhorn Syndrome children are desired. What if, for whatever reason, people wanted Wolf-Hirschhorn children? People got pregnant and hoped against hope that they fell into that 1 in 50,000. "Oh, wow!" they'd say. "You have a Wolf-Hirschhorn baby! I've never known anyone who has one. You're so lucky!"

I don't mean to minimize the medical difficulties of Wolf-Hirschhorn Syndrome. They can be quite profound. What I mean to do is visit an alternate reality, just for a moment. Fiona's syndrome means that she will probably need some kind of care her whole life. But as a parent, what if that were a coveted position? My daughter may never leave me with the sadness of an empty nest. There's a privilege in caring for her gem of a self. Fiona's syndrome means that she moves slowly from developmental stage to developmental stage, making the whole "They grow up so fast" cliché all but a mystery to me. What if this slow development was viewed positively: a chance to smell the roses, to see in all its minutiae the subtle learnings of a little girl? And as for the hardest, scariest aspect of WHS—the seizures and the consequent risk of early mortality—well that one's harder to turn positive, but what if we respected it as an opportunity to live life in the moment? To appreciate who we have when we have them. And love fiercely until we lose.

You could speculate the same for children with Down syndrome or autism, or any condition for that matter. What if, in the eyes of hopeful pregnant women, these children were the coveted ones? Is it just a mental act in absurdity? A practice in naivety, ignoring the difficulties of any given special need? I don't think so. I think it actually teaches us something. It teaches us to remember that cultural preferences are to some degree conditioned. And it teaches us to see the value in people who are differently abled.

The other day, a friend of mine said she appreciated one of my remarks about things *not* to say to a new mother of a special needs kid. But she also wanted to know, what *should* she say? What helps to hear? It was a fair enough question. At first I didn't think I had anything to offer. Then I remembered the single best thing someone had said to me about Fiona. It was at the start of her diagnosis, when the pediatrician suggested that perhaps she had something chromosomal. And my sister said, "Whatever she has, nothing will change the fact that she's beautiful, and we love her."

Nothing will change the fact that she's beautiful, and we love her.

Those words got tattooed somewhere in my soul, and they carried me forward.

Should you ever find yourself in a position where a friend or family member or even just an acquaintance has a child that most of society would consider "less-than-desirable," my advice is to congratulate them. Do it wholeheartedly. Sure, you can offer them the space to vocalize their grief. But you don't need to grieve with them. Tell them their child is beautiful, and perfect, and loved. Tell them their child is a profound gift to this world. Because it's all true. Though I didn't know any of this until Fiona. Yeah. That's how smart she is.

Torso of Clay
Christy Spaulding Boyer

Awakening

I stand in the center of a utilitarian restroom of stark white. Frozen to the tiles are my brown shoes, the good walking shoes that embarrass me. They look huge and ugly upon my thin legs in navy ribbed tights. Across from my line of vision is what keeps me stunned and transfixed, a teenage boy, his body twisted in palsy, his legs stretched as if pulled by invisible pulleys. He is confined to a chair of black and silver metal, yet his whole body seems to fight in vain to fly. His mother fails to shield him from my hypnotic stare. She is drying his face with a towel.

My mother whispers not to stare, and I hear her somewhere far away in my mind and somehow come back, a gentle pull on my hand. This is my first memory of seeing someone with profound disabilities. I hate this term "profound disabilities." It is heavy, unmanageable, and jarring in its rooted reality. I hate this term, and yet it describes the life my son lived for fourteen years better than any other of the terms that I learned and tested on my heart—but I have no memory of uttering this word. What I did say was his name, "Clay," thousands of times. And I heard it countless times in the people in the Midwestern town who asked sometimes out of concern, and other times out of habit: "How's Clay? How's Clay? How's Clay?" I never once knew how I should answer that question.

Born Drowning

After my son is born a tragic birth straight into breathing aids and resuscitations, briskly moving top nurses and doctors, a helicopter to the Children's Hospital an hour away, with words like seizures and brain injury, I stand in the bathroom of the Ronald McDonald House and stare at myself in the mirror. My cheeks are flushed prettily. Were I to have a husband who loved me, he would kiss that pretty blush, tell me I was brave and strong, I think. My breasts are huge and feel like they are filled with sharp rocks, stabbing from the inside out. The milk has nowhere to go, it bleeds like spreading ink onto my grey sweater. I am fascinated and angry at the beauty of these womanly breasts. Would

130

I have acted and have been treated more like a woman and less like a child if I had had the full breasts? I ask myself. I take lipstick from my purse. I see my brown diary. I see my son, in the future, the teenage boy in the utilitarian bathroom. I tear out pages my brown book into furious shreds. I make them as tiny as I can. I want them to go back in time, to never have even pre-existed, let alone existed at all.

There is a phone call for me from the doctor. "Good news, we removed the ventilator and your baby can breathe on his own. Next we'll try the bottle again."

"What happens if he can't eat?" I ask, hearing my little girl voice echo through the wires. "We'll cross that bridge when we come to it," he answers.

"But what will happen if he can't eat?" I ask again.

"We'll talk about that if that happens," he answers. "We need to know about the father. Is he in any way dangerous?"

Dangerous. No. No, he is not dangerous.

"Can we trust him to visit the baby?"

Can we trust him to visit the baby.

"He is just...unpredictable," I say.

"Unpredictable, how? What do you mean by unpredictable?"

I want to say it is just I never know if he is coming or going, that he is always running, that I never know if he will be here or there, or nowhere or everywhere,

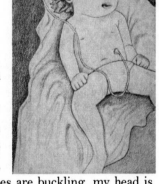

but the world is crashing in on me, my knees are buckling, my head is stabbing, my body is screaming a bladder infection, I am allergic to the penicillin, my stitches are burning, my head is pounding, the iron lid is shutting on my future. "I don't know," I answer. "What will happen if he can't eat?"

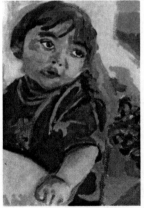

Pastel Portrait

I think Clay was one year old when I drew a pastel drawing of him. I remember debating if I should include the feeding tube in the drawing or not. I couldn't decide which would be more respectful. I decided to leave it in. It was spring, and we lived together in a one-bedroom apartment. Back then, we didn't have a feeding pump, we had a large syringe that connected to the tubing. It had a Velcro strap that wrapped around the top, and a cotton tie, which could be tied or pinned to something above. I poured formula every ten minutes into this syringe and then clamped the tube until the next time. I left the door open to the tiny front porch. Our window faced the side of the house that our apartment belonged to. Across from us was an older couple and the lady spent many hours in her garden, watering, and picking dead buds off of plants. My tiny kitchen had pink and white plaid wallpaper and a mini half stove. We listened to a lot of blues music and NPR. This is where we met my husband, Marc. We fell into one another's arms in a beautiful textured heap. He was a thinker. He watched all the details, how to feed Clay with the tube and the syringe and the formula.

And one day he said, "Can I try?"

And I said, "Yes."

On the Floor

Once I changed my son's diaper on the couch on a bed pad in our living room. I bent over the couch. He was maybe ten years old. His body was completely limp but stiff at the same time. I lifted his legs to try to wipe everywhere that was needed. This was particularly messy. It might take the whole baby wipe box to clean it up. His legs were heavy. I tried to grasp under his knees to lift him up more, so I could clean where I needed too, which was all the way up part of his back. At that moment, I lost grip, and he slid off of the couch straight on top of me and the floor. Shit was everywhere. All over him. All over me. All over the floor. I stared at his pale body, his arms out to the sides and his head turned to the side, looking exactly like a crucified Christ. This seemed like a cruel joke. He didn't react. He didn't cry. He lay there as if nothing had happened. I fell into sobs. I tried to lift him through all the shit, and I couldn't get a grip. The bathroom was a long way off, down a long hallway. My sobs were racking my body, leaving me even less in control. My son was close to my size now.

I finally called my dad. I don't remember what task he had to leave or what he was doing or where he was, but he came over. I had to swallow my pride to call him, but shit had taken over. I know he helped me figure it out. I don't remember how we picked him up or how we cleaned him or how I cleaned myself, only my dad staying very calm and saying something like, "It's okay." Life went back to the way it was, and I kept changing diapers. But that moment is vivid. What was important about it? It was a strong moment, us both covered in shit, me sobbing, Clay looking like the naked Christ spread on the floor. Was it a religious moment? No. Was it a holy moment? No. It was a helpless moment, it was an isolating moment. It was the moment I said, I don't think I can keep going.

The world was going on outside, people were at work, children were at school, lovers were meeting for lunch, and somewhere there were people somewhat like us, another mother with her child on the floor covered in shit, a wife with her husband on the floor covered in shit, a nurse at a nursing home, a daughter with her mother, but our helplessness kept us from being together and saying, "Oh, I'm not the only one!" We had shit to clean up.

Spring Rush

It was spring. Clay was eleven. He lay in his bed while I spoke to my friend on the phone. It was a beautiful day. We had the windows open. The two younger children were playing. Marc was finishing frying the black bean cakes that I had started. He left the kitchen when he heard Clay crying. He called me from his room in what I knew was an emergency. I got off the phone and ran back.

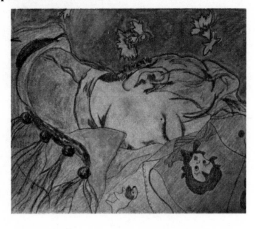

Clay had thrown up something brown and wrong looking. Something else seeped out of his G-tube. And something else ran steadily out the sides of his lips. His face was a horrible shade of gray. Marc and I stood there stunned. He had seemed just fine the day before. We were silent until I said, "I think we're losing him."

"Me too," Marc whispered.

My feet went numb. I couldn't move. Then I could. I walked across the hall and stood in the bathroom. I was trembling. I walked back in his room.

"We need to call the doctor," Marc said.

I said, "He's not going to....at some point he..." I couldn't get the words out. "Are we supposed to just let him..." I started.

"That would be neglect. I'm not letting him die of neglect," he choked back.

I watched my husband pick up our boy, and it was unbearable. Marc whisked him into the van. I watched Clay's bobbing pale face race down the sidewalk as Marc pulled his chair. The sky had gotten darker. I stayed home with the other two children. We didn't know what they might see. I didn't sleep all night. I stood by the phone. I cleaned the entire house. I tried to rehearse words for what we would tell our four year old. I could not come up with a single combination of words that would work for our four year old. Marc called. Things weren't good. We were losing him. I trembled and trembled and trembled, and my feet were as cold as ice for hours. I never slept that night, and the next day my dad and I drove the two babies to Riley Hospital, thinking it was goodbye. But it wasn't.

Painting of Ophelia

Though it wasn't the first time I had seen a copy of the painting, it was the first time I had spent a good amount of time staring and staring at it. At first, all I could see was its beauty, its peacefulness, Ophelia's relief. But, then I was haunted all night long. Ophelia was in my dreams, my subconscious, behind my eyes a lot. I woke with a racing heart, drenched in sweat, more than once. The water was murky, I couldn't see what was in it. It was horror. I was horrified that I loved the painting so much. The image is meant to be the moment right before Ophelia dies. That lingering spot.

My son was eleven, and for that many years, I had been told he would live for this much longer or that much longer, that I should prepare myself. It had formed in my mind through this experience that he lingered there in that tender spot between life and death. Did he really? I don't know, but it's what my mind did with the circumstance. And so I lingered, and I lingered on the lingering. And the haunting of the lingering, because that's the thing about lingering, it lingers like a ghost. Lingering is slow motion. Or even a stand still. And it is tender, too tender for much of the world. The world says: "it is too sad, too haunting, too weird." Eventually the world says, "Don't you have some place to go? Something to do?" My son was haunting. His skin was ghostly white. He had circles under his eyes. His eyes often rolled back into his head. He was stiff and rigid. He moaned loudly in the night. When my middle son was four, he said, "Mommy does Clay think he's a ghost or something? He sounds like a ghost. He's white and he sounds like a ghost."

I wondered once, why, when I was stuck in the street with his wheelchair in the snow, why the bus pulled off and no one offered to help. Why there were several cars in the street waiting for the bus to pass, and they all stared at us struggling, but no one got out of their car and offered to help. Did they not care? Then I thought perhaps they thought they would hurt our pride? Was that it? Then I thought, were they afraid of us? Horrified by us? Did we look too frightening and freakish to them? I don't know.

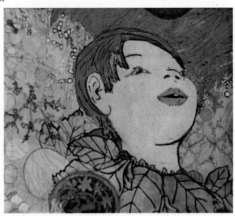

The world said to us, "Don't you have some place to go? Don't you know what's going on in the world?" No, no, we said, we're still here, lingering here where the world stands still. The busy world sped past us. We were still there. That's lingering. We're here. Here. Here, beside this quiet pond. The rest of the world is hard for us to see. There's so much shrubbery, overgrown weeds surrounding us. No, we really can't see past where we lay very well. I was lucky to be there, there where my son and I lingered, not because I was learning how precious life is from my son, not because we were "blessed" with hardship, but I was lucky because he was still there with us. And when a child is your child, you want him here. Even when here is where the water never ripples, and you can't see through its heavy moss. Even when the water looks black, murky, unknown, like something lurks in it. Here is where you want your child. Here. Here. Here. Here. Lingering. Haunted. Here. But this is still not it. What I'm trying to say is an itch right under the shoulder blade. I just can't reach it. I'm speaking of a spot in a shrubbery maze, hard to find, hidden, tiny, secret, easy to miss. A pretty broken Robin's eggshell, holding a bit of yolk, under dried grey-brown leaves of lacy holes, stuffed beneath the shrubs branches. Only a little child, playing in the maze might find it and wonder at its blue beauty, its lost yolk.

The Edge

(*In the hospital room*)

CLAY'S MOTHER

Clay, while you rest and sleep, I am going to read some poetry while I eat lunch in the cafeteria.

(In the cafeteria)

POET

What's going on here?

CLAY'S MOTHER

Well—

POET

I don't understand the clothing you all are wearing today. These clothes make no sense. They mean nothing.

CLAY'S MOTHER

I know. You look lovely though. Your dress is like a painting.

POET

Hmmmm... Those black long cloaks those women are wearing make sense.

CLAY'S MOTHER

I know, but I'm not Muslim.

POET

So pretend to be Muslim then. Or, you could wear all white like Emily Dickenson. Or all black like Johnny Cash.

CLAY'S MOTHER

I've thought of that. It wouldn't work.

POET

Why not? You just don't want to enough. I think today's clothes are distracting. How can you even concentrate on reflecting?

CLAY'S MOTHER

I can't!

POET

You need a nun's habit.

CLAY'S MOTHER

I know, but I'm not a nun either.

POET

So? Don't you think it would be worth it to steal a nun's habit if it could help you concentrate on these thoughts that you're trying to understand? Where are your priorities?

CLAY'S MOTHER

You make it sound so easy. Right. I'll just go steal a habit.

(In the hospital room)

POET

So what is going on here?

CLAY'S MOTHER

My son is suffering. I usually can hear my son. I usually can feel his emotions, sense what he needs, but I feel millions of miles away from him. At least I thought I could hear him. Maybe I imagined the whole thing his entire life.

POET

What does that mean?

CLAY'S MOTHER

I'm so terrified it means he has lost his will to live. I'm afraid we are forcing him to live somehow. This is torture. I am fairly certain that this could drive me insane. It seems that whatever I do, I'm just a horrible person either way. I don't know how to honor him and all I want to do is honor him. It seems absolutely impossible to honor him! The blackness of this unknown sucks me in like a hole. Where is the honor? Honor! Honor! Honor! Where? Where? Where? Where is it? Where is it? Where is it? Where is he? Where is he? Where? I can't find him!

(*POET shows no change of emotion in her face or stance. She is unaffected by CLAY'S MOTHER'S outburst.*)

POET

Did you ever stand on the edge of a cliff, a very high one, over a stormy sea, in the cold wind?

CLAY'S MOTHER

It seems like I have, but I haven't. No, I haven't.

POET

You should. It's the only way to feel alive sometimes.

CLAY'S MOTHER

So that means...you're making a comparison. Let's see...

POET

I'm just saying go do it sometime.

CLAY'S MOTHER

I envy you. Do you see any cliffs around here? I bet you always stood by cliffs in your life, just whenever you felt like you needed to be invigorated. Just, Cliffs. Everywhere. Real Cliffs. Cliffs by the sea. I envy you so much.

POET

Maybe you aren't supposed to do anything but read right now.

(The DOCTOR walks into the room and begins to talk about building up a nutritional pad. CLAY'S MOTHER talks back to him. They talk medical for a few minutes. POET is staring out the window. POET steps in front of CLAY'S MOTHER abruptly.)

POET

I'm sorry, I'm having a hard time with this.

DOCTOR

With...?

(He heard her?)

CLAY'S MOTHER

With...with...with...philosophical questions. Or spiritual questions. Or...
Is there someone I can talk to?

DOCTOR

Well, that depends. There is the social worker. Or the chaplain.

(POET turns back to the window and stares again.)

CLAY'S MOTHER

The…chaplain I guess.

DOCTOR

We can arrange that.

(The DOCTOR exits.)

POET

You and that doctor talk a strange language. You both sound like robots. It's creepy. You don't really want to talk to the chaplain do you?

CLAY'S MOTHER

No, I don't. I thought I did, but I don't know what to say now. I want to read more poetry. Who else should I read? Poet? Are you still there? Oh, right, you didn't come and be my imaginary friend to tell me what poetry to read. Right. Or did you? I do want to go stand on the edge of a cliff, Poet. And I still think you meant something more about that.

Oh, you meant that it is impossible to decide which is more powerful, the sea or the sky, right? They are equal in their grandness?

Or you meant that I am standing on the edge of a cliff, but with-out the sea spray or the wind in our hair, how can I feel real, it that it?

No, you meant that my son is standing on the edge of a cliff but can't feel the sea spray or the wind.

Or you meant that you had cliffs like this all over the place to stand in and feel alive, but how can we feel alive in this hospital, so far from nature, where all the cliffs are metaphorical?

Or you meant, I'm not supposed to do anything, just stand at the cliff and feel everything that there is to feel there, stand beside my son between the sea and the sky and feel every trace of wind and every mini mist of salt water.

Or really what you really meant that there could be a life, an immobile life, a lifetime spent standing still on the edge of a cliff and you could say that this life never went anywhere or you could say that it learned to know the sea's spray intimately and the mystery of the wind by heart.

The Poet has gone, son, and now there are hundreds of people in our room. I've been tripping over Bibles all morning, because the Bible Study group knows what it is we should do about the feeding tube. And the high school debate team has been discussing our situation on your bed. They get too loud sometimes, and I keep getting paper cuts on their index cards. And the judges are still deciding who won the debate. The teenagers are so nervous waiting to see. Two couples are on a dinner date, over pasta and wine on the empty bed beside us. They are having such a lovely evening and quite an entertaining and stimulating conversation about our circumstance just prior to dessert. They know what we should do as well. The college philosophy class is cramped in our hospital bathroom. They are still unsure what we should do, but it certainly has been an interesting class! Some of the scientists know, and some of the politicians, they know too. At this moment, I'm going to ask all of them if they please wouldn't mind leaving and giving us some privacy. It's enough to think about, just the two of us here.

Familiarity

My nana used to blanch tomatoes and peel back their skin for a salad. The result was that the homegrown tomato juice would blend with the ranch dressing and make it pink and would further flavor the lettuce as well. It also made the whole house smell like fresh tomatoes. She used to make a pitcher of sugar water for iced tea, so that we could sweeten our tea without the granules that otherwise wouldn't dissolve in a cold glass. She served this in a small caramel-colored pitcher with dark brown glaze that dripped down the sides so that it looked like melting chocolate. She was a trained vocalist, and everything she said sounded like a piece of a song or a music box that opened and shut. These are the things I miss. I can conjure up these little details in my mind and go back, can sit at her dining room table on a Sunday, hear the chimes on the porch coming in through a cracked window, see the pattern of light the lace curtains made on the pale blue carpet. I can taste the iceberg lettuce salad, the yeast rolls, the simple beef roast with potato and carrot, seasoned with salt, pepper, and Worcestershire sauce. I can hear ice tea spoons melodiously clinking as we stirred sugar water into ice tea. I can hear her laugh like a bell, see my dad yawn rather immodestly, begin to feel sleepy myself right before dessert, rest my head on my hand over my plate.

I long for many things now gone away. There are things I miss about Clay. Even though he was never able to talk or hold his head up or walk or run, there were things he used to. He used to laugh and smile in a way that seemed something holy was taking over his body. I miss when he was small enough that I could hold him in my lap. I remember, back when just him and I lived in a tiny one-room apartment. I would open the door and let the air come in through the screen, then fold up his tight body in my crossed legs and rock in the old rocker that I had bought for $5 at a yard sale. The fabric was torn and yellow foam spilled out, but the pink and brown floral fabric was also worn in a cozy way that made me feel safe. We would rock because he arched rigidly and cried from the discomfort of his tight muscle tone, but eventually he would let go and give in to sleep. I was lonely, exhausted, yes, but I was happy. In many of those moments with my son I thought that he was all I would ever need to keep going in this world.

Eleven years later, in enter my two younger sons, my dad, and I into the Emergency Room at the Children's Hospital. My husband and Clay, now twelve, had spent the whole night there because there is no room in the ICU. The scent of the ER courses through our nostrils and skin. This smell—taste even when it hits your mouth—is a mixture of sweetness, saltiness, chemicals, plastics, sweat, metal, and blood. At the same time, it brings both nightmarish memories and tender ones. The lights are fluorescent and jeering, and the tubes are an obscene puzzle that is beyond being solved. My four-year-old Glen steps in the room and stops abruptly, clearly stunned, though I tried my best to prepare him. I quickly grasp his shoulders protectively. Clay looks awful, my husband stares into space and is clearly on another planet. Staying there all night will do that to you. I brush Clay's hair back from his forehead. How many times had I brushed oily hospital hair from this pale and clammy face? It always seemed like the only thing to do.

"Want to go get him a present?" I say suddenly to Glen.

"Yes," he is sure of this. We are both relieved as we walk to the gift store. Glen picks a small backpack that has stuffed horses hanging from it.

"Clay likes horses," he says.

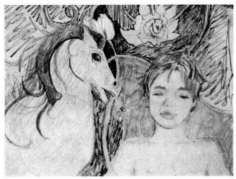

"Yes," I answer, "and we can put it on his wheelchair." This statement quickly turns in my stomach as I realize there might not be a wheelchair anymore.

We take the overly expensive backpack to the make-shift ICU room. On the walk back, there is the usual sad-smile exchange shared with other parents, the "lose-yourself-in-me" aquarium, the Ryan White Memorial of a giant hand, interns clad in tailored black whose fullness of promise makes a literal breeze as they sweep by, then finally the click/swoosh of the giant automatic doors opening to the ER, and the voooom/ SLAM/click/LOCK that followed. It's like entering a vault, or Star Trek Enterprise. Back in the room, I turn off the lights. This is actually inappropriate to do in an ER room, but I've ceased caring.

The next thing that I remember is nursing my youngest, Frankie, in a chair made for tall non-nursing men while trying to keep a blanket over his head, which he didn't want. I gaze into space, as sounds circle my head. There is the beep... beep... beep... ring... beep... the nurses speaking about pizza at the main desk, making jokes, laughing, speaking in crescendos and decrescendos as they move through the hall. The sinks pump on and off next door with a shoom-sha-koom. My dad has his science fiction paperback open, holding it up to the hall light. Marc takes Glen on a walk. Frankie is nodding off in my trembling arms. Clay is asleep.

I am having trouble looking at him. I have the dilemma I've had before. There is a pressure so strong to measure every inch of his physical body. The panic that I'm not memorizing him fully enough makes me want to turn my eyes completely. I have a knot in my stomach. I am still dissatisfied with the lighting. The hall lights are cutting into the room in an unnatural way. There are no patterns in this light. There are no windows in the ER. There's nothing natural in the ER. I know this. I know this. I know this place: the place that pokes and prods the very limits of what we call waiting. I desperately want out of there, as I always do. I know how to want out of the ER vault, how to see the whole place through eyes and skin that long for fresh air, to hunger for a smiling Clay in the sunshine. I almost want to say I know it to perfection. I hate it here. Or do I? One day, I'll desire to be right here where I sit just now. I can't decide. I hate this place. I know this place. I'm familiar with this place, I know its details and more than that there are bits and pieces of my son left in the corners of its cabinets, the smooth cracks of the floor tiles, behind the plate of the light switch. Is familiarity, even for a place like this, worth something? Is it? There goes my chest. It's starting to ache. I just don't want to let him go.

Several years later, I do let him go. His dies in his bed at home one Saturday morning. His familiar shell is carried out of my front door. Now I shall, again, ask myself the question. Is the well-known scent and sight of the hospital worth something? I shrug. Maybe it was, but it is not now. Not really, no, not compared to the familiarity of my son. This life, Clay's life, close and well known to me, leaves me in poignant longing, and asking if it was all a dream. I am grateful that I memorized his frame like a map, but I understand in retrospect, there was no need to work so hard at it. My eldest son is recorded and written down within my inner compass. I laugh wryly at myself, of two years prior, how descriptive I was of a mere room in which my son's breathing body lay. All else in memory fades to grey now, compared to the rise and fall of a single chest.

Water

The day before his death, we know. I give him many sponge baths, drag the washcloth over every inch, in the order that it goes, in the way I have always done. I call Marc and I say he is not doing well and I just know. Come home. What do we do? I ask. We take him to the water, my husband says. We put his chair all the way back. We cover him with a blanket and tuck a pillow onto the foot rest of the wheelchair for his paper thin feet. We take his brothers too. We drive in the van. We cry. We look through the windows to the bright sunny day. It is September and hot because it is Florida. We have only lived here for two months. How will we get him to the water? The chair won't go through the sand and this beach is so long. We carry him, Marc answers. I grab our younger sons' hands. Let them go first, I say. Marc lifts Clay with a grunt and must move fast as the momentum of his weight pulls him forward. I close the lift impatiently before the boys and I run behind them in the sand. I am crying so much I can't see. Everything is watercolor. I know there are people around but they are fuzzy blobs like great balls of colorful yarn. We step around them blindly, my eyes fixed on what seems like a clear golden orb of my husband and my son. Now he has him in the water, where he can stand and hold him floating like a lily pad, moving him back and forth gently and slowly so that his legs swing like a pendulum. We reach them and gather together, our family of five. I can't stop crying. It's okay, my husband says. No it's not, I say. He shifts his balance to support Clay with one arm and wraps my chin and cheek lightly with his other hand. Look at him, he says. Clay's eyes are closed, his curved wrists out to his sides, his legs floating in a frog position, his face only slightly pained. His brothers each have their arms around my neck, their legs around my torso. The water is silver gold. The shimmering of it clings to our skin. It stretches for miles and miles.

Fifteen Years Earlier

We are driving in an Indiana night, between the cornfields under so many stars. The windows are down and I sit in the passenger seat beside this boy, Jonathon. Soon we will conceive a child together. In the backseat is his friend Nathan, a stranger to me, who seems to have some sort of young wisdom that I find fascinating. Jonathon and Nathan pass a roach back and forth.

"Have you ever been in love?" I ask Nathan.

"Yes," he says.

"What does it feel like? What does it feel like to be with that person?"

Nathan takes a long drag, holds it, and releases it to the air of the racing window. "It isn't so much how you feel when you're with someone you love," he says. "It's how you feel without them."

I turn in my seat to better see him. "What do you mean? How does it feel to be without them?"

He coughs, and his voice is lower, entrenched with the pot. "It feels like an ache, but the deepest kind. It is in the pit of your stomach and in your chest, like you didn't know the insides of your body could go that deep. It feels like you aren't whole the entire time you are away from that person, like you don't know if you can live without them. It's like, there is nothing that hurts more than being separated from someone you truly love. Hurts like Hell."

I turn to Jonathan. I look for his eyes. Is this the way he feels? Is this the way I feel? Is this what my pain is, the horrible curdling in my stomach, the sad empty hole in my chest? He is focused on the roach, the wind in his hair. No, I haven't found it yet. But I want it. I want it so much.

The Beginning: Four Pounds, Twelve Ounces
Heather Kirn Lanier

"What a little peanut!" the midwife said as my baby dangled above my half-naked body. Peanut—it was the nicest thing anyone would say about the thing that fast became the focus of my baby: her size. Knee-deep in a birthing pool with my glasses off, I couldn't see my child, and as a first-time mom I couldn't differentiate between small newborn and really freaking small newborn, of which my daughter was the latter. Then the nurses whisked her away, and there was silence, and when I asked if my baby was okay, repeatedly asked, *please, is my baby okay?*, the nurse with me wouldn't answer.

*

But minutes later, our nameless kiddo was on my chest, nose smashed from the squeeze, looking wide-eyed and stunned by the world. All was well, and I was exhausted, and here she was, this person my body knew intimately for forty weeks, but a person I was nonetheless just meeting now.

*

But I could still feel it: the cloud of concern that hung over the room, the nurses' worries, the *why is she so small?*, which spiked my stress hormones and is the reason I don't have a good sense of what mothers mean when they talk about the post-birthing bliss if you go *au-naturel.*

"She's got good tone," said the first pediatrician, holding her in his two hands, inspecting her back. "Her ears are typically set." He kept looking at her. "The question is, why's she so small?"

I was sitting in bed, jamming a chicken salad sandwich into my mouth, reveling in the fact that, for the first time in forty weeks, I was eating a meal without guarding my gag reflex. I was ravenous. It was the best chicken salad on the planet. I didn't have the focus to think aloud with him.

Then he said, "maybe something genetic."

I tried to ignore this. It sounded surreal, foreign, untrue. Too rare. Not my story. Not our family's story. Must be the medical community worrying for no reason. Still, we stayed the night just to be sure she was well.

*

The second pediatrician wanted to know about the placenta. Was anything awry about the placenta? Too small? Not equipped to feed wee Fiona, who now had a name? I had no idea. I told him I'd seen the placenta, and as it was the first placenta I'd seen in this world, I had no idea if it had been a good placenta or a bad one. It looked like a piece of rare meat.

If it's not the placenta, he told me, then it's the baby. "You see," he said before offering a metaphor that every beginning doctor in med school should learn never, ever to use, "It's either bad seed or bad soil."

He meant, either I'd provided ninth months of bad nutrition for my baby, or my child began from a bad seed. Which made her a bad plant.

When he left, I cried. I tried to eat. The lactation consultant tried again to get Fiona to latch. I cried some more.

Then we took our release papers and fled the hospital.

We drove home slowly in the right lane at rush hour, surrounded by fast-whizzing trucks and SUV's, and I sat in the back with my baby. The world seemed too hard and fast and sharp-edged for the softness of a newborn. I did not know then how lucky we were—that she'd had no complications, had spent no time in the NICU, was swallowing her milk, that she was well enough for all the doctors and nurses to send her home, which is not the case for many kids born with her syndrome.

*

Three days after her birth, still stressed by her smallness and the uncertainty of it, we saw our family doctor. He said she was the most alert newborn he'd ever seen. "She's perfect," he said. "She's the perfect size for her!" the nurse agreed. I sighed in relief.

I now consider this visit a blessing: it offered us two months of ignorance, two months of normalcy, two months to see our daughter as a perfect being rather than a series of pathologies to address. Every parent deserves this. I thank God for a doctor's cluelessness.

She wouldn't latch. This became the focus of motherhood. Getting that tiny mouth around the boob. We tried, she refused, we drop-fed her, I pumped. But she ate. Two ounces at a time. And she never spit up. To burp her, I learned to bounce her vigorously. Other mothers warned me at first, then stared amazed at a just-fed baby, bouncing in my hands, keeping everyone's clothes puke-free.

Two months old, she gave her first gummy, wide-mouthed smile. But beneath the fatigue of three and four feedings a night, I still had the nagging feeling. The echo of that first pediatrician's concerns, "Maybe something genetic." The ominous words of the second pediatrician, "Bad seed or bad soil." Tests on the placenta had come out fine. Which left only one other option.

"But the other doctor said she was perfect," a well-meaning family member countered. Still, my husband and I made an appointment for another pediatrician and I sweated it for weeks. I knew something was coming, a shift in our parenting, in our lives.

Thus began the chain of appointments: the pediatrician found the heart murmur. We had an appointment for an Echo. The Echo found ASD and pulmonary valve stenosis. We got her blood drawn. I was convinced she had Turner's. Then Noonan's. Both genetic syndromes that made for small babies and heart anomalies. She gave us her first giggle in the meantime: On September 11. A child of irony.

When the doctor called with the results, my husband, my daughter, and I had a flight to catch in three hours. He said the words quickly while we rushed to get ready. She was missing something on the short arm of the fourth chromosome. To which I thought, *Oh, the short arm. Who needs all of that.*

It turns out that a person who wishes to ever live independently will need all of the short arm of his or her fourth chromosome. But it would take me awhile to realize this.

Instead, all I knew was that my daughter now had a syndrome: something with a hyphen. I couldn't even remember it. My mouth couldn't get around that second word. Hirshel? Hersh what? Without

148

having the time to dive into the internet, we left for a vacation with family, where aunts and uncles and cousins and great-grandparents met her for the first time, held her, adored her, loved her, and nobody said one thing about her seven-pound frame. She was almost four months old.

*

Wolf-Hirschhorn Syndrome. A one in 50,000 occurrence. Rarer than getting hit by lightning. Your odds of becoming a pro athlete are twice as good as your odds of being born with Wolf-Hirschhorn.

"So we have a special needs child," I said to my husband, not really knowing what that meant, not knowing how limited, or unlimited, her life would be, but accepting it. My husband was steering the pram around the neighborhood. Fiona was sleeping. A strange calm descended. A calm I don't always have, but a calm I go back to in the darkest times.

*

And then one night I tapped my fingers hesitantly on the keypad of my laptop and Googled it, her syndrome. It was past ten-o-clock, and I should have been asleep, and all the windows were dark, and the Internet dealt me its cold, clinically-termed blows. I read about the seizure disorders. The kidney and heart troubles. Read the words "moderate to severe cognitive disabilities." Probably read another way to phrase that, but I refuse to type it here. And I read that "some kids even walk and say a few words."

Even. As though a few words and some independent steps are victories. This was before I realized that yes, they are. This was before I could appreciate, could even peek an inch into the seriously heart-expanding life I was in for. Instead, I wept with a kind of panicked, this-can't-be-real fear, the kind that happens only a few times in one's life, that grips you by the throat, that makes it so you think maybe you can't breathe. You probably know the kind of moments I'm talking about— the ground seems to break beneath you, and there is nothing to grasp onto, nothing to steady yourself in a life that is suddenly alien and upside down and what is this? This death of your old way of being? The windows were black, the ground broke, the internet glowed with its surreal bad news, and I was floating in the darkness.

And then I read that we—my husband and I—had a 33% chance of losing her in the first two years of her life.

I went to the kitchen and sobbed, and she was sleeping upstairs, and the sadness was no longer the selfish reaction that my baby wasn't, would not be perfectly able-bodied, but that my baby could suffer, that I already loved her so much my heart broke at the thought of losing her in the next two years.

My husband hugged me and said, "If our time with her is limited, then I'm just going to make sure that I love her the best I can, every day."

It was wise, a lesson I'd learned plenty before. Cherish what you have, when you have it. But it took on a new and imperative meaning now that I was a parent. It did not erase the sorrow, but it offered me a way forward. I wiped my eyes and agreed. She would be our blessing, no matter how long we had her.

*

The geneticist was a delightful red-headed cherub. That's what we called him. The red-headed cherub. He opened a binder, showed us a diagram of twenty-six chromosomes, all looking like overly-xeroxed copies of broken, black ramen noodles. He pointed to number four. He didn't tell us anything new. But he told us in a way that made me feel like this life of Fiona's was just fine as it was.

"A deletion," he called it. Not "a defect."

"A genetic anomaly" rather than an "abnormality."

"Possible intellectual disabilities," he said. Not "mental retardation."

"She'll probably always be small," he said. "She probably won't learn to crawl or walk when other kids do. But we won't put limits on her."

And then he and his superior outlined more tests—kidneys, eyes. They'd start with a swallow study.

The geneticist explained that swallowing was a relatively complex thing. That the mouth has to push the food forward in one way and backward in another way, and meanwhile guard the airway, and this was a difficult cognitive skill. So the greatest risk to Fiona right now, he told us, was swallowing. Could she swallow? Or was she silently choking on her own spit? Many kids with WHS silently aspirate, he told us. This could cause her lungs irreparable harm.

I nodded through all of this, and thought what a feat it was to swallow, and admired all the people I saw walking on the street today who were chatting on the phone and looking at the clouds and worrying about their finances, all while swallowing, automatically, any fluid in their mouths. And rather than bemoan that my daughter might not be able to swallow, I reveled in the amazement that was swallowing, and humanity's overwhelming adeptness at it! We were geniuses out there! All of us! Swallowing!

Afterward, my husband and I took Fiona into the family restroom for a diaper changing, where a floor length mirror was warped on the wall so bad it could compete with a funhouse. "Look at this," he said, all giddy, and I walked over and stood on the adult-sized diaper changing table, and got my head level with his, and saw that his forehead was ginormous and his mouth microscopically small, and my forehead was microscopically small and my mouth ginormous, and we laughed and laughed at the body and the craziness of difference and the okayness of those differences. And I recognized that, from here on out, I'd need this way of seeing.

*

I'd later learn that plenty of parents have not been blessed with such a positive genetics appointment. For a child with WHS, the prognosis was once "doom and gloom," as some parents say. *Your child will not walk, will not talk, will have no personality. Will be a vegetable.* This was what parents were told, and the outdated research sometimes perpetuates, even today. I know parents of three and four year olds— kids who are now saying *mama* and running around at lightning speed—who were told the same. Your child will be a vegetable, they were told. And now they boast on blogs and on Facebook and in person that their kids have defied the doctors.

But my heart breaks for the parents who have to process that kind of news. And it breaks for parents of children who *are* more limited—perhaps nonverbal, perhaps non-mobile—but are still far from "vegetables," a term that is ableist and crude and should never be used to describe even the most disabled of people, because what knowledge do we have to say we know when the divine light bulbs in our beings shuts out? And now I'm ranting. And I'll stop.

I'm grateful beyond words that our geneticist was realistic, nonjudgmental, and open to the many possibilities that Fiona could have in store for us. And that after he asked, "Is this your first?," and after we told him yes, he offered a hearty, "Congratulations!"

*

Everything a parent can take for granted got stripped away. This was not as painful as it sounds. We found ourselves rejoicing at the good news that the ENT doctors relayed: she could swallow her own spit! She could swallow breast milk, formula! She was protecting her airway! After a black spaghetti-like tube had been sent up her nostril and down her throat, and after doctors watched on video the two holes of her esophagus and her airway as she screamed through the feedings, the world seemed eternally optimistic! And it also felt surreal—we were elated over a bodily function most of us take for granted.

But this is our life now. This is our baseline. We rejoice over small things.

That day, we treated ourselves to Eggs Benedict at a fancy breakfast joint. And from then on, I repeat this to myself as a victory, as a reminder of all our blessings: she can swallow her own spit! She has seizures, heart anomalies, low tone, global delays. The list goes on. But her abilities are still mesmerizing. Her kidneys function. Her eyes can see. Her ears can hear. She can laugh. She can love. And she can swallow her own spit! Thank God.

Show & Tell: Part II
Anna Yarrow

5.

My mom doesn't know
how to play my games
so I get mad
and we both go
find a book to read
instead.

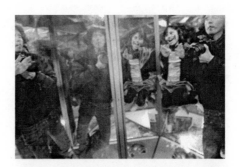

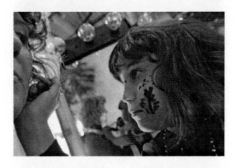

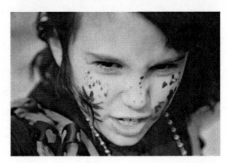

6.

My mom says
I'm the battery
that gets her up
in the morning.
I like telling jokes.
—What did the big
armpit say to the
small armpit?
—Respect your odors!
That's funny, because
I don't respect anyone,
and I *like* going
to the principal's office,
and when I grow up
I'm going to let
my children do
whatever they want!

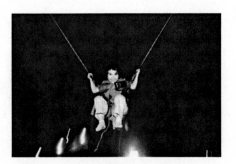

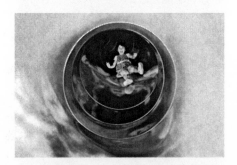

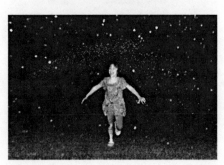

7.

Maybe this life isn't so bad
(Except for hair
brushing/washing/cutting
which is bad, bad, BAD!
In my world
there would be
no hair.)
Optical illusions are cool,
and Oman, where I was born.
I used to ride camels,
and mom swam
with me on her back
to protect me from crabs.

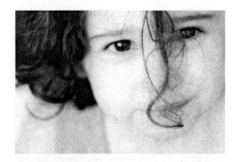

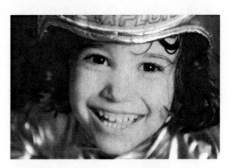

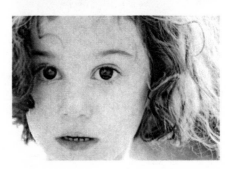

Departing Holland
Deborah Leigh Norman

When my second son was born two months early and later diagnosed with Down syndrome, somewhere in the flurry of reading I consumed, I came across the poem "Welcome to Holland" by Emily Perl Kingsley. Ms. Kingsley describes having a child with a disability like going on a trip to Italy but instead you land in Holland. In my state of confusion and numbness, the words from Ms. Kingsley helped to give a framework to my feelings and much of my mind racing.

The hardest part for me was thinking about what this new member of our family would mean to my first son, then just three years old. I had a mix of fear and guilt for what my older son may have to deal with and for how his life would be negatively impacted. I knew that my husband and I would handle things; we were adults. But for my young son, who had no choice in having a sibling enter his life, how would having a new brother and now a brother with a disability affect him?

Perhaps part of these feelings was the guilt that any parent may go through when they have a second child. The first child's life was going along just fine—did they really want or need a sibling? Most parents probably justify the new addition by thinking that even though the adjustment is hard at first, that the older child will be better off because the child will now have someone to share life with and, hopefully, have a lifelong friend even after the parents have died. However, when we found out our son has Down syndrome, I wondered, would he be able to share life with his big brother and be a friend and confidant? What did this mean for our family? I had a bright, curious, beautiful son—clearly in Italy, and now I had a son unexpectedly in Holland. How could I be two moms in two different countries, speaking two different languages?

I ventured into this new place and met some helpful moms and early intervention therapists. I did not have answers to many questions but, like Holland, having a child with Down syndrome was turning out to be a welcoming and fine place. Holland is beautiful with remarkable architecture, including the canal district. This land of windmills evokes peace and serenity. Holland is one of the world's largest producers of flowers. Just the Keukenhof Gardens alone has seven million bulbs planted annually. The amazing museums, such as the Anne Frank House, are inspiring. Vincent Van Gogh lived in Amsterdam at one point in his life, and the Van Gogh Museum permanent collection has over two hundred of his works.

I understood landing in Italy from my experience with my first son. Italy also has some incredible sites. Pompeii, the Pantheon, the Leaning Tower of Pisa, and the island of Sicily all offer history, scenery, and unique styles. No wonder Italy is one of the top five countries visited around the world with over forty million visitors annually.

Somewhere along the way, however, I realized and, more importantly, I decided that I didn't have to stay in Holland, or in Italy for that matter, and I did not have to choose to blindly travel back and forth the eight hundred and fifty miles between the two countries. The rest of the world is pretty incredible too. I am one mother of two sons, and we are connected. Like the Mississippi River a few miles from our house, we as a family flow through life together on all of its twists and turns sometimes quickly and sometimes meandering.

I have learned best from watching my two sons together. I see that my greatest worry—for my son having a brother with Down syndrome—has turned into the best gift in life and that his little brother has taught him things I never could. They share an amazing connection that continues to astonish me. I see the understanding, devotion and joy that they have most strongly for each other. They have showed me we speak the same language of love and that we will not be kept in separate places.

I have wondered why I feel differently than Ms. Kingsley, and I believe it is because of her. Since she and many other parents worked for better opportunities for their children with disabilities, there is more inclusion and acceptance. Her work and words had a positive influence on so many people.

Through time and travel, I am learning on this journey, and I look forward with excitement and anticipation to where it leads instead of feeling like it is already defined by a diagnosis. In addition to Italy and Holland, I look forward to traveling to Shanghai, the Amazon rainforest, Paris, the Serengeti, and much more.

The Prize
Ann Bremer

At thirty-eight years old, my odds of having a baby with Down syndrome were one in 180. In other words, if you gathered 180, 38-year-old pregnant women in a room, only one would be awarded this life-altering prize. I never win anything, why would I expect to win this?

In the middle of my pregnancy when I received a phone call saying some blood work had come back indicating that my odds of winning were now 1 in 110, I did what any good ostrich would do and put my head in the sand. There would be no meeting with a geneticist, no ultrasound, and no amniocentesis. There would only be the remaining months of an easy pregnancy occasionally interrupted by a new awareness of women at the mall who had been the unfortunate winners of the Down syndrome lottery.

Very early on a December morning two and a half weeks before my due date, I awoke with indigestion, which came and went with predictable frequency. Four hours later, after a harrowing ride through rush hour traffic and an unplanned drug-free delivery, my husband and I heard the words, "It's a boy!"

When they laid my sweet bundle on my tummy, I examined him for signs of Down syndrome. When I saw that he looked like my other babies, I breathed a sigh of relief. But the doctor and nurse spoke in hushed tones, and then the nurse let me know she suspected I was the lottery winner. Thirty minutes later the specialist concurred. My little boy had Down syndrome. I didn't want this prize. Alone in my bed that night, I did what any hormonal, exhausted new mother of a child she didn't want would do and sobbed uncontrollably.

"God chooses special parents for special children," well-meaning friends and acquaintances told me.

Baloney.

Parents of children with special needs don't come to their positions with the talent and temperament required to meet those needs. Like me, they were minding their own business living average lives when they were plucked from obscurity and called to do more than they ever imagined they could. Motivated by a fierce love, they rose to the occasion and earned the moniker "special parents" through hard work, worry, and self-sacrifice. Special parents aren't chosen, they're made.

My son was only hours old when I was presented with a long list of possible medical issues. Forty to fifty percent of children with Down syndrome have heart defects; five to fifteen percent will develop celiac disease; five percent have gastrointestinal malformations; five percent will have seizures; five percent will have hypothyroidism; and one percent will develop leukemia. My son's heart was pronounced good, and his gastrointestinal system was given the all clear after he pooped and peed properly. I assumed there would be no more unexpected statistical anomalies, ignored the list of potential problems, and got down to the business of loving my baby.

Few of my son's needs achieved the status of special, most being of the average variety. As expected, his development was delayed and milestones were missed. What was entirely unexpected was the undiluted joy I felt as his mother. His presence in my life, in our family, killed my aspirations to perfection. With nothing to prove, I felt a freedom I had never before known.

When my son was just two years old, we defied the odds again when he joined the one percent of children with Down syndrome who develop leukemia. Upon hearing the diagnosis, I did what any good mother would do and cursed.

The standard treatment for boys with acute lymphoblastic leukemia is three years of chemotherapy. For three years, I watched as my little boy struggled with the side effects of the poison we pumped into his body to keep him alive. I cried when the drugs reduced my normally sweet child to a crying, screaming mess. By the end of treatment, he was extremely weak with legs like spaghetti noodles, but I rejoiced because he was alive! I remembered the mother who cried the night he was born, the one who didn't want him, and was happy to find I no longer recognized her.

Today my son is ten years old. He likes bluegrass music, chocolate cake, and prefers running to walking. When I was pregnant with his younger brother and sister, I did what any good ostrich would do and put my head in the sand refusing all prenatal testing. But this ostrich was not afraid. This ostrich was well informed, choosing the coolness and darkness of the sand over the heat and bright lights of a world that thinks winning the prize a second or third time would be a tragedy.

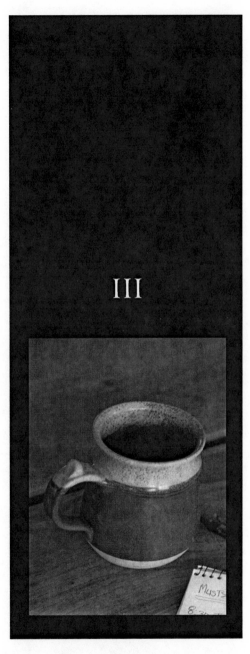

III

"Through all the grief and mourning, joy does come. It always does. It comes with a kiss and a hug. Joy comes with each new word she speaks. It comes when she dresses up in her cowboy hat, boots, and comes out swinging her pretend lasso. Joy comes from watching her love life in the way I sometimes wish I could."   -MaDonna Maurer

My Life Changed
Stephanie A. Sumulong

One of the hardest phone calls I have ever had to make was late in the evening on May 5, 2009. I had to call my parents to let them know that their grandson had been born. That call was supposed to be an exciting one, but at the time, it wasn't for me because I had to tell my parents that the doctors suspected my son, Owen, had Down syndrome. I remember just blurting it out because I didn't think I would be able to tell them if I didn't say something immediately. One thing they said stuck with me—"So? We still love him."

I realized then that even though I was scared, and I had little experience in the world of Down syndrome and special needs, I was going to love that boy something fierce. That love was only reinforced when Owen had to have open-heart surgery at four months old. I'll never forget the feeling of pure fear when I handed him over to the anesthesiology team that morning, not knowing how he would do with the surgery. When he came out better than ever, I knew we had gone through one of our worst experiences as parents and had survived.

Owen has taught me time and again what pure joy looks like and feels like every time he tackles something new and works hard to learn a new skill. I never gave much thought to certain things like learning to write with a pencil, holding scissors to cut, blowing bubbles, drinking with a straw or an open cup, or walking up and down the stairs. These are things I just DO without thinking about the mechanics involved. But in order for my son to do those things, he has to learn each part of the process correctly and then practice for a long period of time before he can have it mastered. I have learned to practice serious levels of patience that I never believed I was capable of because the waiting game can take a long time!

I find joy and pride in the accomplishments that come for Owen, no matter how long it has taken: walking at twenty-six months, using a spoon and fork at age three, blowing bubbles in the water just two months shy of turning four years old. I find that I celebrate these milestones loudly, and I wonder if I would have done that if Owen didn't have Down syndrome. In a way, it makes me sad to think that I wouldn't have been as excited about these accomplishments if he had been a typically developing child. I take more joy in seeing his happiness at doing things for himself than I ever thought possible and each new accomplishment makes me less worried for his future.

There are things about having a child with special needs that don't seem fair: the extra doctors, therapy visits, surgeries, special education process, the red tape in dealing with securing resources or funds from insurance, the constant worry about the future and whether your child will be able to function on his own, the comparison of your child to your friends' typical developing children and the feeling of never measuring up, the feeling that you aren't doing enough to help your child succeed, the nagging feeling you get when things are going well that the other shoe is about to drop, or the loneliness that sets in because most people just don't get what it feels like to be you.

Four years into this journey and I am just starting to feel comfortable with myself, our daily life, and who my son is starting to become. I no longer constantly think about Down syndrome every moment of every day. It's still a huge part of our lives and always will be, but it doesn't control everything we do or everything we think about. More of my time is spent doing things that other mothers of four year olds do—helping Owen learn his letters, numbers, colors, and how to write his name, making messes in the kitchen while baking cookies, finger painting grand masterpieces, and taking trips to the zoo to see his precious monkeys.

My journey has been different, complicated, and exhausting, but I'm still here. I'm trying to pave the road for my son to make his life a little easier. I know we will have bumps in the road, we already have, but I know now that I can handle them, maybe not always with the exact grace I'd like, but we will make it through the tough times just as we make it through the fun times—with love and joy. To say that Owen brings me so much joy is an understatement—the kid radiates pure joy. To feel that much real joy on a daily basis means life is being lived, and I know that Owen's life is definitely worth living.

What Max Says

Alison Auerbach

"That's not what Max says," Gabriel states emphatically, as though presenting irrefutable proof that I am (again) wrong.

"Max is seven years old, Gabriel. I know he's smart, but I'm pretty sure that I have more experience and education than he does. He's not always right." I'm arguing with an eight-year-old about my intellectual superiority over a seven-year-old.

"No one is right *all* the time, Mom," Gabriel reassures me with my own words, spoken over many a math assignment or guitar practice, and adds the standard comforting pat to my arm. "But Max usually is."

There are seven children in Gabriel's class, and he calls his classmates his "six best friends." When I asked once about a "very best friend," he refused to choose among them. My husband and I have learned to ferret out the identities of Gabriel's favored playmates by noting the names that come up most frequently in his conversation. When I started hearing Max's name over and over, in stories about everything from science experiments to Lego-building, I knew that it was time to program his mom's number into my cell phone.

Sure enough, their teacher soon begins to refer to them as the Dynamic Duo. The day that they cover a cardboard box—and themselves—with glue and straw building the first Little Pig's house, I dub them the Gruesome Twosome. I know very little about Max beyond this outstanding ability to make a mess: He is charming, but this obvious to anyone who has ever laid eyes on him. His mop of strawberry blonde hair is so eye-catching that a passer-by once asked his mother if she dyed it. Wide blue eyes and a pointed, elfin chin complete the picture of childish innocence, right up until he flashes a mischievous, freckle-framed grin. When asked for details about Max's likes, dislikes, family, and so on, Gabriel says only that he is "really cool," and they spend most of their play dates in the basement, away from prying maternal eyes.

Just when I'm seriously considering grilling Gabriel's teachers to learn more about Max and his friendship with my son, I discover that the boys are enrolled in the same specialized summer camp. The commute to and from this camp is a misery that involves driving the city's worst-designed expressway in the height of rush hour. As happy as I am that Gabriel loves the camp and will have a good friend in his group, I am ecstatic that I get along well with Katie, Max's mom, and that they live on our side of town. Because that means we have a carpool.

The best thing about carpool, of course, is that I won't have to make the horrible drive twice a day, five days a week for six weeks. The next best thing is that carpool is the motherlode of information gathering: The kids tend to forget that there's a grown-up in the front seat. A quiet driver who listens carefully can learn all sorts of things about her child and his friends.

As it turns out, it takes less than five minutes on the very first day of camp to learn that Max's freckles and wide eyes belie a sense of compassion and empathy well beyond his seven years.

That day, as I'm gathering my purse and cell phone to head out the door, I notice that Gabriel's backpack is no longer on its hook. Then I notice that Gabriel is no longer in the house. Just before I panic, I see the open door out to the garage and flip on the light. My son is already buckled into his seat, backpack on the floor in front of him.

When he sees me at the door, he flounces impatiently, "Come on, Mom! Max is waiting!"

"All right, Big Shot. Let's hit the road."

On cue, Gabriel chimes in as has become our tradition. Pulling out of the garage, we sing together, "Hit the road, Jack, and doncha come back no more, no more, no more, no more! Hit the road, Jack, and doncha come back no more!" Aretha Franklin can relax—neither Gabriel nor I will be challenging her rule as the Queen of Soul.

"Hit the road Jack, and doncha come back no more. Doncha come back no more. Doncha come back no more. Doncha come back no more. Doncha come back no more. Doncha come back no more. Doncha come back no more..."

"Dude, is your needle stuck?"

"What?" Oh, that's right. No one born in 2002 would catch a record player reference.

"You're stuck. On the song."

"No I'm not."

"Okay, you're not." I've had this argument enough times to know it's not worth having again. We ride in silence toward the YMCA, where we will rendezvous with Max for the trek to camp.

"Doncha come back no more. Doncha come back no more. Doncha come back no more. Doncha come back..."

And yet the record player comparison is apt. Gabriel's euphoria over going to camp with his idol has short-circuited the switch that controls his neuronal "needle," leaving it stuck firmly in one of his favorite songs. This repetition is one of his few recognizably "autistic" behaviors. Once Gabriel's primary method of communication, the behavior has largely disappeared thanks to time and therapy. But when he's feeling anything—excitement, anxiety, even amusement—very intensely, it's almost as though his brain is too overwhelmed to operate speech and thought at the same speed. In these moments, the repetition returns, perhaps involuntarily or possibly as a way to calm himself.

"Doncha come back no more. Doncha come back no more. Doncha come back no more. Doncha come back no more..."

"Gabriel, it's a long ride to camp, and I don't think I can listen to that song all the way there. Do you think you can stop?"

"Yeah. Can I sing until Max gets in the car? Then we can talk about Mario!"

"It's a deal." Interesting. Gabriel seems to have connected the repetition with his eagerness to see his friend. That's a new awareness for him that I file away for future reference.

We pull into the YMCA parking lot, and I slide into a space next to Katie's car. Max bounds out of his mom's car and into mine. I'm not sure his feet actually touch the ground in between. Katie is a few steps behind, slowed by the weight of Max's backpack, lunchbox, and car seat.

"Hi Gabriel! Hi Ms. Gabriel's Mom! What's your name again?"

Before I can answer, he and Gabriel are deep in conversation about camp and Mario, and I turn my attention to helping Katie with all of his gear. After all the hugging and kissing and buckling and settling, we're finally ready to take on the expressway. True to his word, Gabriel has stopped singing now that Max is in the car, and I'm enjoying this rare glimpse into my son's social life.

"Who's your favorite Super Mario character, Max?" Gabriel bounces in his seat, he's so excited to have someone else who cares about Mario in the car.

"You know! It's Luigi!"

"Mine's Toad!"

"I know! But why do you like him so much?"

"Because he's awesome!" cries my son. "Awesome, awesome, awesome!"

Max laughs. "Luigi is triple awesome too!"

Gabriel is enchanted by this new phrase. "Triple awesome, triple awesome, triple awesome!" he chants. "Say it again!"

Max, delighted to have an audience, happily obliges, "Luigi and Toad are triple awesome!"

"Say it again!"

"Luigi and Toad are triple awesome!"

"Triple awesome, triple awesome! Can you say it again?"

"OK. Luigi and Toad are triple awesome."

Lather, rinse, repeat. I can tell by the note of exasperation creeping into his voice that Max's enthusiasm for this conversation is starting to flag.

"Gabriel," I get his attention.

"What Mom?"

"It's enough, Buddy," I say as gently as I can. "You've said it three or four times now. It's time to move on."

Gabriel considers this, replaying the last few minutes in his head to see if I am right. (God forbid he ever just take it on faith that I know what I'm talking about.) While he thinks, Max leans forward.

"It's OK."

"Pardon me, Max?"

"I said, 'It's OK.' I know that Gabriel repeats stuff sometimes. It's no big deal."

"Yeah, Mom," my son chimes in. "It's not a big deal or anything."

Just like that, the intensity of the moment abates, and the repetition disappears.

"Thanks, Max," I reply quietly. "Gabriel is lucky to have a friend like you."

"I am," Gabriel agrees, though he has no idea just how lucky he is.

"Awww. Well I think Gabriel's pretty cool too!"

Bright as Max is, even he doesn't yet understand how valuable he is to my son. If Max had made fun of Gabriel for repeating, snapped at him to stop it, or otherwise indicated that the behavior was somehow "wrong," Gabriel would have been devastated, as the idea of getting anything incorrect terrifies him. Instead, Max framed the repetition as something a little different, something unique to my son, but not wrong or bad.

Gabriel will eventually have to learn how to handle intolerance from his peers, and the only way for him to have the self-respect to weather it is to recognize that "different" isn't right or wrong. It just is. While I can tell him this every night for the next ten years, that won't penetrate nearly as well as the acceptance of a good friend. Max gave Gabriel two gifts: acceptance and a concrete example of how one should expect to be treated by a friend.

168

Max *is* the superior intellect in this car. This scabby-kneed mud magnet of a boy actually stepped into my shoes for a split second, unprompted. He instinctively knew to reassure *me* that he is at ease with who Gabriel is. The hair on my arms stands up as this clicks in my brain.

With a friend like Max in Gabriel's life, I might worry just a little less about my son getting teased for his social immaturity. I might let myself hope for more for Gabriel than simply not being ostracized. One day I might even be able to expect it.

Your Eyes, My Daughter, Are Genius Caliber

Heather Kirn Lanier

I spot the five-pointed star inside your iris,
blue aquatic, like a chunk
of the cartoon heavens sought a long, enduring swim.
Your gloss-black pupils reflect
my ceasing furrows, my stressed brow
easing into adoration. I see you
seeing me—mother struck
by the ancient wonder: what
impossible mathematics
in the molecules of your seeing.
A brain to move a hand to swipe my hair.
Ears to catch the peripheral
hey, and you turn to face
a face your mind already mapped—the giver
of food, love. And all your vowels,
riper than fruits in our wooden bowl,
your oohs and ahs and ehs
whole as grapes in your tiny mouth. They say
you don't meet your milestones.
That the arm of one chromosome
has a hiccup in its copies.
But you are living. You sense. You suck
your thumb. You receive
the world, your awareness like daily haiku.
This morning's message
caught your eye a long infant-minute
and I thought you were zoning out
on window light, or worse, seizing. I got down
to your level and saw it too:
a wind chime glimmering
against the suburbs' winter scene, the brass
tubes lit gold by a low sun. *See it*,
your staring said, that star
in your iris dazzled by the dance.

His Name is Mikey Joe
Sharon Hecker Kroll

Recently, I was in the checkout line at the supermarket with Mikey and his brother. As the teenage girl was busy scanning our groceries, Michael leaned over, grabbed her hand and chirped to get her attention. He has always been a sucker for cute girls. She looked up and smiled as he blew her a kiss. The girl looked at me and asked his name.

My son, Matthew, spoke up and said, "His name is Michael, but we call him Mikey Joe."

I smiled as we left the grocery store. Matthew was right.

Hearing Matthew speak those words took me back to the time when we found out I was pregnant with a boy. I vehemently told my husband, "I don't want him called Mikey."

Tom and I had finally decided on the name of our unborn son. His name would be Michael Joseph and he would be called Michael. We both liked the name Michael, Mike was okay, but we unanimously decided we didn't want him called Mikey. Mikey reminded us of the old Life Cereal commercial where a group of boys were gathered around a table with a new box of cereal. The boys looked upon the cereal with dubious curiosity. It contained no pieces of chocolate or sugar coated flakes, and no cartoon characters were drawn on the front of the box. One boy even quipped, "Hey, let's get Mikey." I remember the younger, gullible brother brought to the table to eat the cereal because he'd try anything and usually hate it.

I did not want my son identified with such a gullible, vulnerable character who would do anything a person asked him to do. Tom and I had thought long and hard about a suitable name. A strong name like Michael would allude to great things. Michael Joseph was to be his name. Michael because it was a strong male name that meant "who is like God." We chose his middle name, Joseph, because that was my husband's uncle's name, and its meaning "God shall add." Not that I felt my son would be a god, but I thought that his name would honor a life filled with promise and expectation.

We were two educated adults who had successful careers and were absolutely giddy with excitement at this new direction our life was taking. Our son was going to be loved and nurtured. When people would talk about him, the words smart, athletic and compassionate would be brought up in the conversation. We predicted that he would possess tenacity and integrity.

The pre-natal vitamins were taken every morning with a glass of water instead of the coffee that I had given up long before I conceived. I was reading the book *What to Expect When You Are Expecting* and knew what to expect at each new stage in the pregnancy. At one of my first appointments, the doctor's tagged my pregnancy, "advanced maternal age." This was due to the fact that I was thirty-five, and in their eyes, I was older than what was optimal for a healthy pregnancy. When did I get so old?

I had all the usual tests, appointments, and ultrasounds, which I passed with flying colors. Despite my age, the pregnancy was progressing smoothly, and Michael was growing in my womb. During a routine check-up and ultra-sound at 30 weeks, my pregnancy veered off the normal, predicted course. The technician was unusually quiet as she focused on Michael's head measurements. She quietly got up and told me that she wanted to get the doctor. The doctor came in and silently looked at the ultrasound. The greenish glow from the machine reflected on his concerned face.

Slowly he turned to me and said, "I am concerned about your son's brain development."

Michael's brain appeared smaller than normal. As he spoke these words, my whole life changed. My feelings of happiness of our antici-pated baby's arrival quickly dissolved and were replaced with emotions of fear, anger, and disbelief. At this moment, I wished that Tom could have been there so we could have faced this together.

As I began to cry, the doctor turned to me and said, "You need to be strong for your baby," and left me to digest the news.

I hated the doctor's callous manner. Later, I would realize the importance of being strong for the battles ahead.

However, at the time, as I digested the news, I became angry with God. Why did it have to be his brain? Why couldn't it have been something else? Michael could have lived without some of his fingers or toes. I would gladly give up an appendage to save his brain. I was having these conversations with God in the hope of bargaining and changing Michael's destiny in life. Even with the birth of my next son, Matthew, I would first ask the doctor about his brain development and remember to count his fingers and toes as an afterthought.

The doctors starting using new names to describe my son: microcephaly, hydrocephalus, and atrophy. What did this mean? As he continued to grow, a team of doctors monitored his brain development.

Several weeks passed with more complications including pre-term labor and bed rest. Finally at thirty-six weeks, Michael was born in a crowded room filled with nurses, perinatologists, neonatologists, pulmonologists, and neurologists. They whispered words of lung maturity and brain bleeds. To the doctors, he was a patient with names that included prematurity, microcephaly, atrophy and a host of others. To them, he was not Michael Joseph, strong and fearless.

Once he was born, more names became associated with his medical condition including apnea, bradycardia, and hypotonia. During his first few weeks of life, the doctors were busy ordering CT scans, MRIs, EEGs and EKGs. More names I needed to understand and accept.

These were not the names I wanted to hear, but ones I was expected to quickly learn if I was able to take him home and care for him. I was told that there was a great chance that he would be developmentally delayed and cognitively impaired. Two more names I was forced to digest.

When the doctor's deemed he was ready, we nervously took him home. We came home equipped with all the typical baby equipment: diapers, car seat, and stroller to name a few. Additionally, we also came home with monitors, medicines and a CPR flow chart to hang on the wall next to the crib and the mobile I had joyfully picked out during the first few months of my pregnancy when life was perfect. A medical dictionary was placed on the bookshelf next to baby books to understand all the new names assigned to my baby. In all of this medical chaos, no one had shown me how to change a diaper, how to swaddle him, or how to breastfeed. How was I going to manage?

That first year was a blur filled with tests, therapies, and doctors' appointments. Entries in his baby book consisted of appointments and therapy schedules, not the notations of goals achieved such as grasping, smiling, rolling over, sitting, crawling and walking. On his first birthday, we propped him up in the high chair and celebrated his special day. There would be no videos of him standing and toddling over to his parents or squealing with delight. Still, we reveled in the fact that he was alive and had expanded our family by one.

The years went by with more news about Michael's development. He would probably never talk, might not be able to feed or dress himself, might not walk, would remain childlike and require full-time care. Our days became consumed with therapies and surgeries to prove the doctors wrong. After two long years of therapy, Michael started taking his first steps. It became our goal to have him walk into the pre-school classroom on his third birthday.

By the time Michael was able to attend pre-school, we had another child in tow. After many meetings with the school district, Michael was ready to go to pre-school. On his third birthday, I showed up at the classroom with cupcakes and a double stroller. I took Michael out of the stroller and set him on the ground. Then I put the cupcakes in the stroller and told Michael's younger brother to stay put. All of Michael's classmates had already run into the classroom, eager to start the day. Now it was Michael's turn. I positioned Michael upright in front of the classroom door. His teacher was kneeling on the floor waiting for him to enter. Michael took one hesitant step and then toddled, with a swagger all his own, across the room's threshold into the outstretched arms of his teacher. His walk was similar to a toddler's first hesitant and unbalanced steps with his wide-based gait and out-stretched arms. It was not attractive, flawless, or accomplished, but he walked! To this day, I can remember, with clarity, the smile on his face and the feeling of my heart bursting with pride.

Many more years passed involving surgeries, multiple trips to the emergency room, and countless hours of therapies. We have all grown in ways that were first impossible to imagine. The whole family has learned signs to help Michael express his needs and desires. Pictures, signs and the old standby of taking us by the hand and showing us what he wants, has helped ease the frustration of being non-verbal.

Nineteen years have gone by. There have been many ups and downs in our lives. I have experienced deep anguish at the direction that his life has taken and great joy when he smiles. We have even attached another name to him. I can't tell you when exactly Michael became Mikey. Somewhere tucked between doctor visits, school meetings and life we eased into the name. Mikey seems like a fitting name for him. It is a suitable name for a person who will always remain a child. Mikey will never drive a car, never go to college, never get married, never have children and never say my name. This development corresponds with all the names linked with Mikey's medical files.

He has grown into a teenager who is taller than me, but still sees the world through child-like wonder. He loves watching the wind blowing through the trees on a spring day, the bright sunshine glistening on freshly fallen snow, flags fluttering in the breeze on the 4th of July, the rippling of water when a stone is skipped on a pond, and the crunching of fallen leaves on the ground in the fall. He can sit in front of the window watching the birds at the birdfeeder and laugh at their antics. Michael doesn't care about titles, material possessions, clothing labels or whether we are on time to our next scheduled doctor appointment.

Our whole family has changed with the birth of Mikey. Many of our so-called friends disappeared after Michael was born. Now, our friends are much smaller in count, but they are true friends. They have been there during the ups and downs and even though they may not understand, they are willing to listen. It has been hard to hear heartless comments spoken about our son. Sometimes such comments are whispered by strangers or blatantly stated by acquaintances under the guise of concern.

Tom and I wanted a child who was smart, athletic and compassionate. We've embraced the gift that he is and are able to see that those dreams have come true. Michael might not be smart by the typical academic definition, but he knows what is important to him. He quickly learned the location of the store that contains helium filled balloons. Despite which direction I am driving, he knows when we are close to this store and demands that we stop. What allows him to know this? Whatever the trigger is, my heart dances with joy when I buy him balloons and see his delight with the bouncing objects that he tries to swat with his hands.

He knows when to look for the big flag flying over the car dealership when we go into the city for his doctor appointments. For a child who is unable to read, how is he able to point to the EXIT sign, look at me, and sign "please" when we are in the long mazes of the hospital halls waiting for a doctor's appointment, lab work, or test?

Some people wouldn't call Mikey athletic by any stretch of the imagination. However, living in his world, we realize that he is fascinated with sports. He loves watching football, basketball and hockey on TV and going to sporting events around town. The sound of the buzzer, the squeak of the shoes on the gym floor, the slap of the puck, the bounce of the ball, and the gymnastics of the cheerleaders all provide entertainment for him. When the scoreboard lights up with fireworks after a goal or basket, he grabs my hand and points to the display with a huge grin on his face.

He has a love for bowling and bowls several times a week. Perhaps Mikey enjoys bowling because he is around all of his friends who are laughing. Maybe it is hearing the ball echo as it rolls down the long wooden path before crashing into the bowling pins. Whatever it is, he gladly gets into the car on bowling nights. By far, his favorite activity is swimming in a pool and not having to fight gravity for a short moment in time. A perfect summer day is floating in the pool, listening to the music and watching his dogs take a flying leap into the pool to fetch the ball that he threw. The bigger the splash they make, the more he laughs.

I don't know how Mikey learned to be compassionate. It isn't anything that was taught, but it is something that is inside him. He gets upset if he sees a baby crying, and looks on with concern if he overhears an argument between two people. He wants everyone to be happy. However, he does have an opinion of who he likes and doesn't like. Usually he and I agree on this topic. I now judge people by how they treat Mikey. I have always wondered, was that his opinion too, or was he just mimicking my feelings? That is one of the questions I will ask him when we meet in Heaven.

Our younger son, Matthew, has also developed these qualities from being around his brother. Even though he complains about home-work and learning, he realizes the gift that enables him to do well academically. No books could teach him such lessons about compassion. However, he shows us each and every day the lessons he has learned by living with Michael.

Matthew also loves to play hockey. By being present for Mikey's countless therapy sessions, he realizes how easily the sport comes to him. This knowledge makes Matthew want to be better.
Mikey is his biggest sports fan and finds nothing funnier than watching two boys slam into the boards on the rink.

Many years have passed since he first toddled into pre-school. We have attended fifteen years of case conferences and developed new Individualized Education Plans (IEPs) to address the goals and challenges of each year. Last year, much thought was put into having Michael attend his high school graduation ceremony. With a graduating class of almost 900, a lot of planning was needed to assure he would be able to make it through the whole ceremony. The day finally came and he was dressed in his cap and gown and seated in his wheelchair, since navigating the long procession into the gym and across the stage would be too exhausting for him.

The ceremony started with the acknowledgement of multiple awards including honors for academic achievements, excellence in sports, and trophies for the accomplishments of the quiz bowl team, spelling team, marching band and orchestra at the state finals. Each of the students accepted their awards with pride in their achievements. The speeches from the salutatorians followed the awards. Their eagerness to graduate and leave home to become independent adults was reflected in their voices as they spoke of the future. During this litany of accolades and promises, a deep sadness enveloped me as it became obvious, once again, of all that Michael would not accomplish in his life. Over the years, the disappointments in his life and development have decreased as we accepted his limitations. However, on this day, the pain was foremost.

The last part of the graduation ceremony was the presentation of the diplomas. Directions were given from the superintendent to postpone cheers and applause until the last child walked across the stage and received their diploma. This was done in an effort to facilitate a speedy delivery. I looked down at Michael on the auditorium floor and wondered if he would be able to sit patiently and quietly through this whole process. I was also wondering why we had him attend this ceremony when it was painfully obvious he really wasn't graduating with his peers. He did not know the meaning of this ceremony and would only receive a blank folder, which should have contained his diploma if he was truly graduating alongside his fellow classmates. As the procession of the students paraded across the stage, Michael, with his paraprofessional, wheeled closer to the stage. He disappeared briefly from our sight as he went behind the stage to get on the wheelchair lift to take him up to receive his diploma.

I was filled with trepidation knowing thousands of people would be watching him go across the stage. Would he scream and babble, would he flap his hands in excitement, or would he sit calmly, quietly and wait his turn, as one of his goals each school year had suggested. I was so nervous that it took me a minute to realize what was happening when they called his name. It started out as a small noise, which exploded into thunder as the whole auditorium was clapping for him, despite the instructions prohibiting this behavior. At first I thought it was the parents in the audience who were clapping for him. However, it became apparent that his classmates led this applause. One by one, his classmates on the auditorium floor stood and applauded as he received his empty folder. I think Tom and I were the only ones in the audience who were still sitting as we were trying to contain our emotions.

What started out as a day of extreme pain, doubt and wondering why we were even there, turned into one of immense pride and pleasure as I realized his student peers also saw him as a beautiful and significant child of this world. Michael was able to transcend all of the different groups in high school. Each of these individuals were able to see his gentle happy demeanor as he passed them in the halls each day smiling and blowing them kisses. Despite their varied dress, diverse hairstyles or individual interests, he never spoke an ill word about them, made fun of them or ignored them. Instead he accepted them for who they were, and they returned the favor.

As we grow older, we are starting to look to the future. The years of sadness and disappointment are mostly gone. Humor has taken its place. Tom and I have both figured out from Mikey, it is better to laugh than cry. We can laugh at his antics and our dysfunctional lives. However, we aren't laughing at him, we are laughing with him. Much like a ten-year sober alcoholic can laugh at a tale of drunkenness.

Our house now contains my burgeoning collection of files and books, all containing names that were unfamiliar to me many years ago. Books titled *Children with Epilepsy*, *The Special Education Maze*, and *The Art of Sign Language* now fill the shelves. All of the baby books were passed on to expectant mothers with the silent prayer that they would find joy in their child no matter what the outcome.

Even with the name Mikey, he is not the gullible child that some might assume. If anything, his strength has changed me. He has taught me to enjoy the simple things in the world, to find the happiness in a different path that was taken, and to love unconditionally. And yes, his name is true to its meaning "who is like God." Mikey is life-affirming, non-judging, and loving of all people. So yes, I have a son, and his name is Mikey Joe.

Tough Love

Robin LaVoie

"Now I've been hangin' around you for days
But when I lean in, you just turn your head away…
I always have to steal my kisses from you
Always have to steal my kisses from you."
—Ben Harper & The Innocent Criminals

I torture my child on a fairly regular basis.

Every time I indulge in this behavior, my son's screams of aggravation and my husband's entreaties to "stop being so mean" convince me to back off, and I am able to refrain for a few days.

But soon enough I am at it again. I can't help it. I tell him, "I am a mom, this is what we do."

And, "You are my son, and I will kiss you if I want to."

Oh, he *hates* that.

Most days, I am very sensitive to the fact that my child is, well, sensitive. His allergy to affection is not just a new pre-teen embarrassment thing. Like many people with autism, my son's sensory system is on high alert, and there is something about a kiss that really rubs him the wrong way. Perhaps my lips feel like sandpaper to him. Or maybe it is the sound of the smack that makes his skin crawl.

My son is so repulsed by the idea that he responds with a frustrated "Ouch!" when I simply *blow* him a kiss, not to mention when I actually touch my lips to his skin. When I do sneak in a quick peck, he grunts "No!" and often hits himself or vigorously rubs the spot where the kiss was planted.

If I really feel like sharing the love, I will give my husband a kiss when my son is in the room. My kid will drop whatever he is doing to run over and give his dad a tap on the head, just to set things right, while giving my husband a very clear look of *you're welcome.*

So, with due respect to my child's aversion, I usually offer appropriate accommodations. I make do with a ruffle of his hair or a squeeze of his hand. I substitute crazy tickle fights for quiet cuddling on the couch. I give my child "deep pressure" squishes instead of gentle hugs. If my kid is in a good mood, I can attack him in a game of "Mommy kisses!" and we laugh as he fights off my maternal advances.

I know that I am lucky to have these interactions with him—some people on the spectrum avoid any kind of physical contact—so I try to keep my kisses to a minimum, no matter how much I crave a tender moment with my child.

But sometimes I just forget. His infectious laugh and beautiful grin bring out the worst in me. When he is upset, I really screw it up. Even after almost fourteen years of parenting this kid, I still try to offer a shoulder rub or soft hug when he is crying. To him, my actions provide the exact opposite of comfort but that maternal instinct to reach out and physically embrace a despondent child is *strong*. I am still learning that my needs and his don't always match up.

My unrelenting displays of affection are not just about what I need as a mother, though. I torture him for his own good. Just like crowded grocery stores, dental exams and public bathrooms, there are things in life that you just have to do—no matter how disgusting and uncomfortable. My rigorous campaign to expose him to these awful and painful obligations in life—including receiving a kiss from someone you love—will ultimately pay off. After years of practice, my son loves the grocery store, successfully endures the dentist, and stresses about the public john a lot less than I do myself.

Someday, his wife will thank me.

And, on those days when it is clear he cannot tolerate any violations of his personal space, I oblige him. I adjust and adapt. I bide my time. I enter his room, ninja-like, after he has fallen asleep. I fix his blanket, so his feet don't stick out. I touch his arm, push his hair away from his forehead, and take in his calm, unworried face. He would probably be horrified to know that I am here, every night, ever so gently stealing the kiss that I cannot give him while he is awake.

I know. I'm so mean.

Joint Attention

Liz Main

My third child was well into his second year when I become aware of his utter indifference to me. He had been so passive up until then, so "easy," that I was frankly delighted with him. I could stay or I could go; he did what he pleased, whether it was spinning the wheels of a Thomas Train or peeling a crate of Clementines I'd left within reach.

If he was thirsty, he'd try to get a drink out of the refrigerator. If the TV frightened him, he would try to turn it off. He didn't see me as a vital middleman, let alone the center of his universe. Other toddlers compete with siblings, telephones, and computers for their mothers' attention—he didn't seemed to notice where my attention lay. His self-absorption was convenient, but it was a fool's paradise. He couldn't flourish like that, and neither could I. The rest of the family was affected as well, particularly his older brother, who was treated more like an object than the solicitous playmate he longed to be.

At two, my son received twenty hours a week of in-home therapy from New Jersey's Early Intervention System. Before his diagnosis on the autism spectrum, I had never given a conscious thought to the way individuals share focus on people, objects or events, a process known as "joint attention." Helping my son develop that ability would soon occupy most of my waking hours.

My son was fortunate to receive applied behavioral analysis (ABA) as well as occupational, speech and physical therapy, but it was Greenspan's Floortime therapy that brought him out of his isolation. It wasn't easy. I had to enter his world to find a way to share it with him. It took time to slow myself down enough to see what he might be looking at. So often it seemed to be nothing at all. But when I let myself see deeply, I might notice a shadow that had captured his attention. And then I let it capture mine as well. We built a close relationship over the draining years I spent engaging his attention second by second, prolonging the moments when we were focusing on the same thing.

When you live with the fear that you will never know your own child, intimacy becomes its own reward. Indeed, my appreciation for the privilege of knowing another person spilled over to all my relationships. I heard my preteen daughter's snarky remarks with new ears that understood her implied question: do you see things the way I see them? And I felt tremendous satisfaction when I realized my other son and I habitually touched base with a glance.

Sloppy though it may be, communication is the way humans connect. So as my son began to look at me and to speak, every interaction was cause for celebration. One night, as I returned home with the kids from one of my daughter's activities, I noticed a full moon. I took my son from his car seat, held him close and pointed to the sky. I recited the long-memorized poetry of *Goodnight Moon.* I looked at him.

"That's the moon," I said, pointing again. I looked back at him and then to the sky. "Moon," I repeated.

He looked at the sky, and then at me. He pointed his finger.

"Moon," he said.

I cried. It was one of the best nights of my life.

My son, now ten, still points his index finger in the precise way he was taught through ABA. I see his outer fingers curl inside his thumb, and I hurt for the painful days my family has shared. When I became a mother, I thought love was the glue that held a family together. But small, intimate moments forge the tightest bonds. If not for my son, I might never have known.

My Daughter Meets the World
Michele McLaughlin

It should be simple enough; people have been doing it since the beginning of time. You have a baby and then you present your baby to the world. You start with your immediate family, your friends, and then you continue to expand your circle. It shouldn't be so complicated, and yet, it seems as though when your baby is born with Down syndrome, even the process of presentation can become delayed.

My daughter was born prematurely, and she was born quickly so no one was the wiser when she came into this world. There wasn't time to call family or friends to let them know. I didn't even bring my camera or a bag to the hospital. It was just supposed to be a quick visit to make sure that everything was fine. The doctor thought it would be best to be checked out by the maternal assessment center, but she was pretty sure I was just experiencing Braxton Hicks contractions.

By the time I got to the hospital, my daughter was trying her best to come out and meet the world. The hospital staff asked me not to push, not to present my baby just yet. They said that people from the NICU needed to come, that they needed to be there for the presentation to make sure all was well. The NICU staff arrived and my daughter was more than ready. After she was born, she was whisked away to an adjacent room while I got increasingly agitated. I mean, I had read all those books that say a baby needs to latch on right away to successfully breastfeed, and I definitely wanted to successfully breastfeed. This was my first baby after all and, like most first-time mothers, I wanted everything to be just right.

My doctor kept going over to the door that opened to the room where my daughter was being poked and prodded and looked over. She was trying to keep it open. She seemed to know that I needed some kind of connection.

She kept saying, "It is just so good to hear a baby crying, to hear that all is well."

I mumbled my agreement, but I really felt like I wouldn't know that all was well until I got to hold her.

The people from the NICU kept closing the door until finally, my obstetrician went into the other room to see what was going on. This woman who had said to me after my triple screen, "There's no way you are having a child with Down syndrome" disappeared into the other room. Moments later, she had to come back and give me the news, "The people from the NICU believe your daughter may have some markers that are consistent with Down syndrome."

I don't think I really even registered the words she was saying because all I WANTED to hear was, "Here's your daughter." I just wanted a chance to hold her, for heaven's sake, but it seemed that wasn't going to happen just yet.

I was put into some sort of recovery area, and it seemed that everyone that passed through would keep trying to assure us over and over that tests to confirm a diagnosis of Down syndrome needed to be done and that they would check more as they were able, etc., etc., etc. until my husband finally looked straight at the woman who was presenting her findings and asked, "Have you ever been wrong with a diagnosis of Down syndrome?"

She seemed to bite the inside of her lip and finally blurted out, "No."

And, I swear I could feel the whole room breathe a collective sigh of relief when my husband responded, "Ok. She has Down syndrome. What now?"

Now to do what should be natural with a new baby, right... present her to our family, our friends, our communities, and the world. But, I delayed. I was worried how people would respond when we presented her and how could I know how other people would react when I hadn't even figured out how I was reacting myself. I felt like I was having what people referred to as an out-of-body experience. It was only slightly less surreal when I finally got to hold her, to meet her, to let her know that I was there. I watched myself take care of this baby, my baby, and then I started reading.

I read book after book. I found many of the stories from other parents of children with Down syndrome helpful and others not so much. There was a story that stuck with me about being in public. The author of the piece described how she initially felt as if people were judging her baby because they would keep staring. She described how she felt like a momma bear and would get very protective until one day, she realized that people stare at ALL babies. They are just so compelling to most of us. It made me wonder what it would be like to have people see my daughter, this child of mine who I was still trying to figure out myself. Would they see an adorable baby? Would they see her diagnosis? Would they be drawn to her or repelled by her?

Since there was only one way to find out the answers to these questions, it really was time to present my daughter. First, I called my family and then my friends. Everyone seemed to react in nearly the same way I was feeling, happy to have my baby here yet confused by what this Down syndrome thing meant.

After discovering that no one in my family was going to disown us and that none of my friends was so repelled that they didn't want to associate with us anymore, I felt better about venturing out into the community. When the people stared, and they did in fact stare, I was ready to chalk it up to "that's what people do with babies because they are so compelling." People were drawn to my daughter right away. I discovered that the people that did notice the extra chromosome only did so because they knew someone—a child, a sibling, a distant relative, or someone else who had Down syndrome.

It actually opened up myriad conversations. I got to ask many people about many things that had been weighing on my mind, most of which boiled down to just one thing... how are they doing? I wanted to know if the thirty-five year old was living on his own, if the twenty-one year old had found a job that she liked, if the sixteen year old liked her classes, if the nine year old could read, if the two year old was walking yet. I felt unbelievable relief to hear other people's stories about their sister with Down syndrome who had just gotten married, their son with Down syndrome who had been specifically sought out for a particular job opening, their neighbor with Down syndrome who was driving a car, their student with Down syndrome who was homecoming king, their cousin with Down syndrome who loved his new apartment.

I continued to be drawn to families in this Down syndrome community, families I likely never would have known in any other way. I connected, my daughter connected, and I kept presenting her to more and more people.

She continued to grow and attended several preschools where she was presented to many teachers and many more classmates. There was a teacher who honestly wasn't initially sure if she even wanted to have my daughter in her school at all. She was definitely hesitant. But, once I presented my daughter to her, she decided to give it a go and then she spent countless days of that year telling me how "typical" my daughter seemed. The best part though, occurred at the end of the school year at a family picnic. My daughter was climbing on the play structure at the park with her classmates and one of them stopped dead in her tracks as my daughter was following her up the steps to the big slide and looked at her so sweetly and so sincerely and said, "I'm really going to miss you next year!"

At other parks and playgrounds, my daughter would inevitably find the people who had worked in special education or who had some kind of a connection that I couldn't see. My daughter would run off along a path near the playground and grab the hand of a woman walking with another child and a dog. I would go after her, and by the time I arrived to apologize for the intrusion, my daughter had firmly presented herself, and the woman was happy for the intrusion she didn't even know she wanted.

So very many times I would watch as someone would be snapped into the present by her wave or greeting. People who were clearly mulling over things that had happened or things that needed to be done would suddenly be given the gift of being present to connect with my daughter even for just a moment. Their faces would lighten and they couldn't help but smile at this little girl raising her hand lightly to her face and wiggling her fingers at them as if she was trying to sprinkle pixie dust. She would say "hi" and sometimes launch into such crazy stories that I would come collect her so that they could get back to their lives, with a new smile on their face.

At the farmers' market my daughter went up to a table where there were beautiful, hand-made forks and spoons carved from wood. She said to the woman selling them that she liked one of the forks, and she picked it up and started to walk away with it. Of course, I had to tell her to put it back and explained that she cannot take things without paying for them. The woman, however, had another plan. She decided that my daughter should have one of these forks that her husband made if she liked them and so she offered one to her. And, when my daughter thought a different one might be better and maybe a spoon would be good too, the woman smiled broadly and gave her all she asked for. So now my daughter has a wooden spoon and fork, and I hope that woman still has a warm memory.

Once on a field trip to a sports arena, my daughter saw the cotton-candy vendor with the giant clouds of sugar on an enormous stick, and she decided this was someone she should know. She went over to him and asked politely, "Can I have one of those, please?"

Even after finding out that she didn't have the money to buy one, without missing a beat, the man very conspiratorially said to my daughter, "Yes you can, but don't tell my boss."

I'm sure this came out of his pocket, but he wanted to give what he could to my daughter.

186

Even while shopping, my daughter found a way to introduce herself to a worker stocking shelves. The worker was passing her time doing her work, and my daughter was passing her time waiting for me, so they were left with time for a conversation. They ended up with such a sweet bond that when my daughter proclaimed that she really wanted some stuffed dog attached to a bucket of treats, the gal stocking shelves took it from her to go to the cashier, she bought it, and then presented it to my daughter.

Don't get me wrong; it is not always candy and roses. Sometimes people are not quite as welcoming as one would hope. Honestly, I think it is like that for all kids at times. But one thing is for sure; there is no standing on the sidelines with my daughter. We are all in. My daughter will make you take notice of her if she wants to get to know you. If you are looking down at the ground in a pensive stare and she decides she needs to meet you, she will cock her head to the side and stick her little face under yours until you are just forced out of your head even for a brief time, and you are given back this present moment. Sometimes she will just say, "hi," and move on leaving you to smile and ponder what it was that had you so fraught with worry or concentration just a moment ago.

People seem to pause and take note of things they might have just rushed past normally. She gets them to appreciate a moment no matter how small. She gets people to see the flower, see the plane, see the puppy, see some joy they might have missed. She gets them to see her. She is good for them. She is good for me. She is good for you. So, world...I present my daughter.

Much is Given
Jamie Pacton

When I was a girl,
my father told me over and over:
"To whom much is given, much is expected."

This mantra followed me
through high school classrooms,
into boggy wetland cleanups and antiseptic nursing homes.
It haunted me in college,
where I was mediocre on my best day.
It's the demon that lies behind all my adult aspirations.
But, it wasn't until my child with autism arrived that I understood it.

Much is given.
In Liam—non-verbal, violent sometimes, just 5 but often far, far
away— I am given too much to handle.
1825 sleepless nights and counting.
Arms covered in bite marks and bruises.
Hips arthritic at 34 from carrying the strain of these early years with
him.
Tears, again and again, that sneak up on me as this life with him
stretches, world without end.

And much is given.
My self.
My words.
My time.
My energy.
My hope.
My heart.
My youth.
I give, and I give, and I give.
And I still don't know what to expect.

He gives too.
Laughter at dawn.
A quiet nuzzle under my arm.
A flash of understanding.
A babbled conversation that tells me how he really feels about
vegetables on his plate.
A kiss on his younger brother's head.

A grinning dance to music that we both love.
A lightness and otherness that reveals
just how crucial his presence is to our family landscape.

Others give much too.
Therapists who teach Liam the same things a thousand, thousand times.
Grandparents who ease our days through gifts, packages, and trips to
Sam's Club.
Friends who wrap their arms around our family because we know now
how to ask for help.
Strangers, who look askance, but embrace my explanations.

I take nothing as a given on this journey,
but much is expected.

Sound, Noise, Music
Alison Auerbach

"IT'S LOOOOOOOUUUUUUUD!" shrieks Gabriel.

We have just stepped from the empty sidewalk into my nine-year-old's favorite pizza place. Ten or twelve diners are chatting quietly, their conversation accompanied by the unmistakable clinking and crashing of an open restaurant kitchen. The background music is classic rock, and our entrance is punctuated by a particularly passionate percussion solo. To me, the noise level is quite tolerable. Certainly not as bad as say, Target on the night before Christmas.

To Gabriel's ears, with their auric nerves intricately rewired by autism, we might as well be sitting next to an amp at a KISS concert. He tries to cover both ears and simultaneously drag me out of the restaurant, becoming frustrated when he realizes he doesn't have enough hands. He settles for using his body like a sheepdog to herd me toward the door, with his hands clamped firmly over his ears.

Thankfully, Savvy Mom, the one who is patient and understanding and doesn't care about the stares from the other diners, is in the house this afternoon. When Tired Mom is running the show, Gabriel's herding generates a power struggle that typically ends in threats or tears. Savvy Mom remembers that the transition from outside sounds (more distant) to inside sounds (much closer) is the hardest part. If we can make it through the next 5 to 10 minutes, keeping panic and anxiety at bay, his ears will adjust enough (like your eyes do when you've been in a darkened room for a few minutes) that he'll be able to enjoy his pizza.

I put my arm around him and walk with him the few steps back to the front door. Kneeling down, I motion for Gabriel to ease up on his ears enough to hear me talk. He lifts all but one finger from each side.

"I know it's hard for you when we come in from outside," I begin.

"YES, IT'S LOUD!" he insists.

"Right. Remember that when you yell, or use your outside voice, everyone else has to talk louder and the noise gets worse, right?"

"YES! I mean, yes."

"Good job. Do you remember how we did this last time? You kept your hands over your ears for just a couple of minutes, and then just your fingers, like you're doing now, and eventually your ears adjusted."

Actually, we've done this the last five or six times we've been here. So far, Gabriel hasn't yet reached the point where he can remember his coping skills through the shock of the noise. He'll get there—I've seen it happen in other situations.

Eventually.

"Oh yeah," Gabriel remembers, and I can see his forehead relax as he also recalls that the noise won't be this intense for the entire meal. He lifts the remaining fingers about a millimeter from his ears, testing. "Hey, it's not loud anymore!"

Just like that, the crisis is over, and he skips over to "his" table, located away from the front entrance (flies might try to eat his pizza), near the bar television (so he can check the baseball scores), and in good proximity to the bathroom (so that he can attack his pepperoni as quickly as possible after washing his hands).

I need a beer.

Actually, what I need is three weeks lying on some tropical beach, possibly with my husband, definitely with a bottomless margarita. But the beer is the best I'm going to get tonight.

Once Gabriel has wrestled off his coat, arms flailing, he tries out each seat at the table. Unlike Goldilocks, he's not looking for the most comfortable chair, but for the best vantage point to watch the TV over the bar. He can't miss a minute of the day's sports scores scrolling across the bottom of the broadcast, though they repeat over and over for at least 30 minutes.

Just as the scores begin their crawl, the kitchen crew cranks up the music. Someone is a heavy metal fan. I flinch and rise halfway out of my seat, expecting Gabriel to run screaming from the restaurant. He doesn't even blink. Safely seated and plugged into ESPN, he's in his zone, impervious to the cacophony blaring through the room.

Someday, I promise myself, I will figure out how a boy rocked to his core by restaurant chatter can tune out Megadeath cranked up to eleven.

In my more honest moments, I admit to myself that I will never figure it out.

*

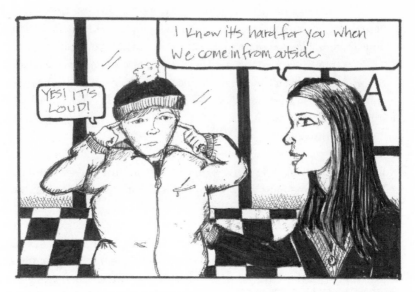

Bridgette Shively

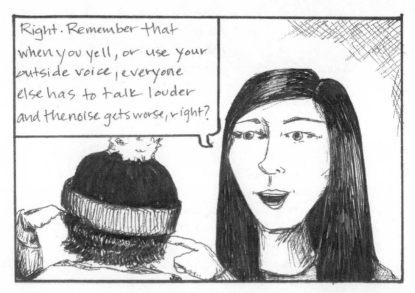

Bridgette Shively

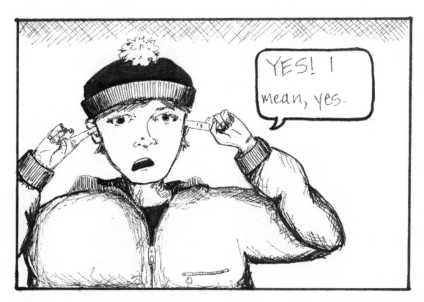

Bridgette Shively

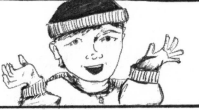

Bridgette Shively

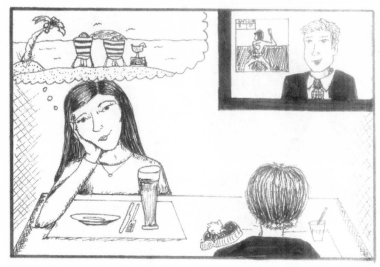

Bridgette Shively

*

"Has he ever played before?"

I startle to attention, jolted away from my animated game world. Without my supervision, Krebl, the game's tiny bug protagonist, knocks a huge boulder on top of himself and dies. Again.

"I'm sorry?"

"Your son," repeats the guitar teacher, with the patience of someone used to working with young children. "Has he ever played the guitar before?"

Yeah, right, I think. Since this is Gabriel's first lesson, this man has no idea that while other preschoolers were swinging T-ball bats or practicing ballet positions, Gabriel was in therapy learning how to talk and figuring out how his fingers worked.

"No. He's been to music classes where the teacher has played, but he's never had lessons or anything. Why?"

John, a tall, reserved man with a slight foreign accent, grins suddenly. He pushes long, graying dark hair off his forehead. "I've never seen anything like it. He remembers all the finger positions after seeing them once and what notes they are. Most kids, it takes them weeks to learn what he just did. Do you or your husband play an instrument?"

I laugh outright at that. I played piano for six years and can barely manage to plunk out "Mary Had a Little Lamb." And the only evidence of Ted's seventh grade battle with the clarinet is a single blackmail-worthy photograph. "No," I manage to choke out around the giggles. "We sing with Gabriel, because he likes music and learns well that way. But if there's any musical talent in the family genes, it skipped several generations."

We both glance over to the subject under discussion, who is perched on the edge of the worn leather waiting-room sofa, fiddling with the tuning pegs on his brand-new guitar.

"I'll have to get you to fix that before we leave," I admit sheepishly. "I have no idea how to tune a guitar."

"He does," John says quietly.

"What?"

"The tuning. He saw me do it when we started the lesson, and he just did it too."

It's what I think of as a savant moment. Autistic savants demonstrate skills that seem like superpowers: Stephen Wiltshire, an autistic architect, can draw whole cities from memory after one flight over the area. This is what most people think of when they hear the word autism, and lots of these people feel free to ask me what my son's "trick" is, as if he's a trained circus animal. As far as I'm concerned, Gabriel's greatest accomplishment to date is learning how to play with a friend without my supervision.

But I have to admit, if we're stuck with the sensitivities and challenges of autism, we might as well get something cool out of the deal. Certainly I often feel that life owes my son a little something extra. So when he taught himself negative numbers at age seven and started to beat me at chess at age nine, I admit that I bragged just a touch.

But all that turned out to be a blip on the radar compared to this musical ability. Because Gabriel's innate guitar talent turns out to be just the beginning of the story.

A few weeks later, my dad is visiting when Gabriel decides to copy the pre-recorded songs on his mini-keyboard on his guitar, having learned the notes by ear.

"Does he have sheet music for those songs?" my dad asks me, wide-eyed.

"Nope."

"So how does he know what note to play on his guitar when he's copying the song?"

"I'm pretty sure he's doing it by ear."

The music has stopped. Turning, I see a Cheshire Cat grin plastered across my son's face. While Gabriel has no idea just how unusual his abilities are, he does have a sense that he pulled off a good trick—and impressed Grandpa.

"I heard the notes on the keyboard songs, Grandpa. That's how I know them," and he bops back into his playroom to continue learning "O Come All Ye Faithful" via electronic sample.

My dad goggles after him for a long minute, then turns back to the conversation. "Is he getting the notes right, do you think?"

"Hell if I know. It sounds right to me. He tunes it, and his teacher says it's right."

My father stops mid-step. "He's tuning it with no comparison? By ear?"

"Yep."

"So it's not just that he can hear a note from the keyboard, and copy it. He's hearing the note in his head?!"

"Yep."

He turns around again, and we lock eyes. "Jesus."

"Yep."

Soon after, my father buys Gabriel a CD featuring the highest and lowest notes each instrument in an orchestra can produce. The notes are not named, only played. As my father plays each example, my son matches the note on his keyboard. When a note is outside the keyboard's range, Gabriel tells his grandpa how many octaves past the end of the keyboard that note would be.

My son's musical ability and his extreme noise sensitivity are opposite sides of the same coin. Gabriel hears things that we neurotypicals (the au courant word for people not on the autism spectrum) don't. The wiring from his ears to his brain is different from ours, and he experiences sound, noise, and music in a way that we can't begin to understand. (Though that doesn't explain why hands that struggled for years to control a pencil can glide so easily over guitar strings.) Someday, I hope, someone will figure out a way to help people on the spectrum filter out the painful auditory input from that which is beautiful and useful.

Perhaps, with enough encouragement and just the right therapies, my son will be the one who figures it out.

Beautiful Smile
Michelle Odland

Weekday afternoons are my favorite time. In the afternoons, I park our minivan in a stuffed elementary school parking lot and cross the basketball court to stand on the sidewalk by the playground door. I'm with a handful of parents and older siblings that pick up their Early Childhood students. We stand by the big yellow school buses and dodge teachers and aides that assist three to five year olds with various disabilities, personalities, and social skills. I stand along the brick wall

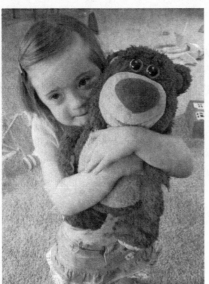

just outside the door, waiting for my own sassy five year old.

I see the smile first through the glass doors: this big grin shows off her dimples and the crinkles in her blue eyes. It is here that I can see her belly move as she giggles and hugs her bear. Her brown bob swings as she hops over sidewalk cracks and her red Yo Gabba Gabba backpack hugs her teeny shoulders.

"Hi, beautiful girl!" I say as is our routine and lean down to get my hug.

She giggles, signs "beautiful," and wraps her little arms around me. She wraps her legs around my waist during the hug, and I settle her on my hip as she holds onto her teddy bear.

"Mu-hah" is the big kiss I give her cheek. "I missed you! Let's go home."

She giggles again and pecks me softly on the cheek. Her little arms squeeze my own, and I can't help but peck her again. I then carry her to the van, because she doesn't like the business of the parking lot, and I don't want to give up that hug.

Our days are not always that way. My Nyssa has Down syndrome, and we have our challenges. If she doesn't want to do something, she'll go limp like a wet noodle and absolutely refuse to move. Forty-five pounds may not seem like much, but she is far stronger than she looks. Like many children with Down syndrome, she is delayed in some of her development. I've never worried about her not being capable, but some things just take her longer. She didn't sit until ten months. She began to walk at three. She still has not mastered pedaling the tricycle.

Speech is her biggest weakness. She has some words: she can name her family, common objects, and can say some colors and shapes, though not all her words are clear. She knows baby sign language and the name of her favorite foods. I'm "Mama," my husband is "Dada," her brother "Na-ton," and her sister is "baby Anna." When she's tired, hungry, or just in a bad mood, she forgets any of her words and gives a loud "meehhhh" to represent what she's thinking. Sometimes I can figure it out. If not, she'll plop her little body on our kitchen floor and yell louder. If frustrated, she'll swat at whomever is near her, which means that she will be angrier as the consequences mean a longer wait.

Some days, I'm so incredibly frustrated by our lack of communication, so tired from breaking up the fights between Nyssa and her sister, that I'm thrilled to get them packing and in the van to school. But when I tell Nyssa it's time for school, she thinks it's hysterical to run down the hallway and try to hide from me. I'll call her name, and she yells, "noooooo!" as she ducks into her bedroom. She'll be sitting on her bed amongst her two stuffed bears and pink flowered blankets when I walk in with a pair of socks.

"It's time for school now." She usually uses her hyperflexibility to pull her feet up to her ears and then kick down on me while yelling something in gibberish to me. I try to patiently remind her that it's time to put shoes and socks on, so we can go to school. If I'm lucky, she'll then plop down and assist me by signing shoes. I then have to squeeze a jacket on her before the little one opens the door to go to the van. (She loves trips, "buh-bye.") I have to follow her and buckle her into the car seat, so she doesn't go down the driveway to the sidewalk. Of course, this means I have to go fetch Nyssa again. And if I'm still lucky, she's actually waiting. More often than not, it's more fun for her to run down the hallway and pull off the jacket and shoes that I just had on her.

When she's finally in the van, we need dancing music. Nyssa has an eclectic taste in music and will dance if she likes it and yell in protest if she doesn't appreciate the song. The ride is only fifteen minutes of dancing and singing.

198

She's happy when we get there and is ready to walk to her classroom. She sits in her "work chair" with her teddy in the nearest chair and attacks her drawing, stamping, or tracing. I get a quick "I love you" sign back, and we blow kisses. I then relish the silence while her sister naps and Nyssa is at school. I know that it won't last long as within a couple hours we make the trip back to school to pick her up.

But then, I will have that beautiful girl smiling at me. Because no matter how our day went, it's all forgiven with a smile and a hug. And my heart melts each time I see those blue eyes crinkle and those tiny little arms squeeze me tight. Even better yet, sometimes I hear "Luh-ooh" with that sign.

Skye Won't Wear Shoes

Ellen E. Moore

(Playground)

Skye prances tippy toes through the wood chips,
climbs the jungle gym with a plush mouse
clutched in one hand, reaches the top and shakes
her head in the breeze, eyes closed, fists clenched.

If you ask her to play, she'll look away
eyes to the ground, but she's fun
to chase, runs and cuts corners, ducks
under, waits till you see her then
swings over and through.

If you ask her a question, she might
not answer, but she'll sing you a tune
while she shows you the moon or
follows a bird song or a plane hum
as it passes through the afternoon sky.

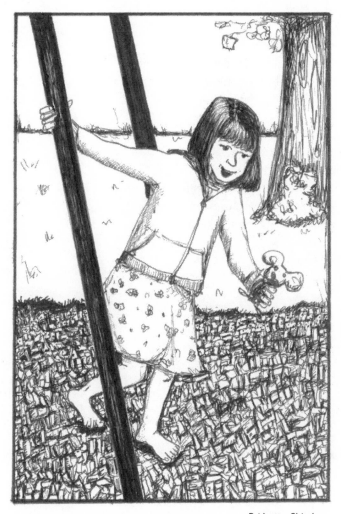

Bridgette Shively

(Dance Class)

While the other girls file into the studio and change
their shoes, barefoot Skye approaches the barre
and the mirror, an arabesque on her toes then
lets go with a twirl and a leap–sashay, sashay,
tour jeté.

The teacher arrives and it's time
to get in line. Her mother presents
her shoes. Skye darts, but her mom cuts
her off at the doorway. Skye closes her eyes
lashes out, pummels her captor in the chest.

Her mom holds her arms and gives her
a choice: We can leave
or you can wear
your ballet shoes. Skye
wears shoes for
exactly forty-five minutes
on Tuesdays.

She's not the best student, follows two
steps behind, till the techno music
from the big girls studio clashes and
Skye turns inward, locks her legs and rocks
out to her own cosmic concert.

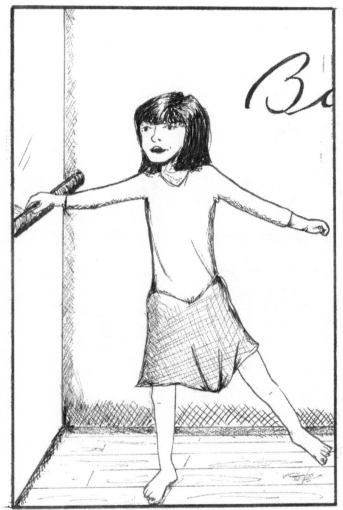

Bridgette Shively

(At Home)

In her own backyard, her trike sits idle
while she swings—"higher" she demands,
"keep pushing." Then abruptly stops.
She climbs to her perch in the honeysuckle tree
rests in the branches, strips off a length of bark,
holds it to her eye, dangles it
up down up down up down.

After bath time, she bounces on her bed while
counting to 100 then asks to be squeezed.
She's wrapped in a tortilla of blankets and
compressed amongst comforters and pillows

till she's ready to settle down and end
her day with stories and kisses
and lights out, like any other
little girl in the world.

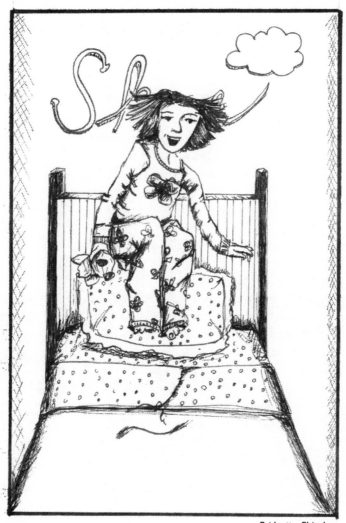

Bridgette Shively

Waiting, Still Waiting for Words
Cynthia J. Patton

I was still in bed when Katie slipped past, heading for the stairs. My slender, caramel-haired daughter didn't look at me or speak. She was a shadow, receding with the dawn.

I huddled beneath the down comforter, filled with foggy, nameless emotions. I knew I should go downstairs and engage her as the specialists had instructed me to do. Make good use of our precious free time. With an autistic child there's always something to work on: social skills, sign language, speech. Instead, a prayer rose unbidden. Please, please give me the words. I can do without hugs and kisses, but I need more words. I need them like air.

Katie was five yet spoke like a two-year-old—when she spoke at all. A knot lodged between my shoulder blades. What if conversation never came? Like most parents, I'd assumed friends and conversation were a given in my daughter's life. I took them for granted until the awful day when Katie was diagnosed with autism spectrum disorder and all those assumptions turned to question marks. Katie was smart enough, but speech remained a challenge. While other parents complained about constant chatter, I longed for it. My daughter's mind was a secret garden, the thoughts overflowing with nowhere to go. I wanted to hear her stories, her emotions, her feeble attempts at jokes. I wanted her to look at me, smile, and say Mommy.

Was it so much to ask?

I released the breath I hadn't realized I'd been holding. I curled around the comforter, golden as a sheaf of wheat. My tears rained down as I prayed for the day the words broke free, flooding fallow fields.

Katie was nonverbal for two years, eight months. At three, after a year of intensive speech therapy, she had a spoken vocabulary of 50 words. By four, she used two-word phrases. By five, she assembled short sentences.

Special needs parenting is often a strange blend of gratitude, sorrow, pride, and guilt. I was excited and proud when Katie mastered a new sentence. Yet I was sad she had to work so hard and guilty I wanted more. Why couldn't I simply be grateful? I was, but it's hard to watch your child struggle, especially when there's nothing to do but wait. For me that's one of the most difficult things about parenting a special needs child—the endless waiting.

At six, Katie answered simple questions. By seven, she used adjectives and worked to master possessive pronouns. I fought for additional speech therapy and finally the long, slow slog ended. Her speech began to gain momentum.

Or maybe that's what I told myself to make it through the day.

One night shortly after she turned eight, Katie asked for the blue dolphin as she climbed into bed. Her words were crystal clear, so I praised her as the speech therapists trained me to do. She asked again, and then again, growing frustrated.

The frustration I understood all too well. "I don't know what you want."

"I want blue dolphin."

I held up a beanie baby. "Do you want the blue cat?"

"No," she said. "Want dolphin please."

"How about sleeping with the cat? You like him."

"No thank you. I want blue dolphin."

"We don't have a dolphin."

"I want blue dolphin." She enunciated every syllable as if I were hard of hearing.

"Katie, we don't have a dolphin." I was struggling to keep my cool.

"Dolphins swim in the water."

"You're right," I said. "They're good swimmers."

Suddenly I had a flash of inspiration and reached into the basket that contains her stuffed animals. "Do you want the lobster?"

My ex-husband and I bought her this toy in Maine after spending a week on Cape Cod. She was eighteen months old, and it was one of our last vacations as a family. It took me a long time to look at the lobster and not get choked up.

But now it's just a lobster. It's also an animal, like the dolphin, that swims in the water.

Katie smiled and reached for the toy. She played with the pinchers while I felt smug about discovering the glitch where her brain veered off course.

She looked up. "This is red. Red lobster."

"I know, but it lives in the water."

Her pained look said I was the one with the neurological problem. "I want blue dolphin."

"Katie, we don't have a dolphin."

She clenched her teeth—the beginning of a full-blown tantrum. I thought fast. "Why don't you pick the animal you want to sleep with?"

This wasn't the routine, but after a long pause she rolled out of bed, rooted around in the basket, and yanked something out. I laughed when I saw Eeyore. "That's not a dolphin. It's a donkey."

"Blue donkey," she said, climbing into bed.

I know Katie knows the difference between a dolphin and a donkey. Sometimes her brain scrambles the words, the same as in the aftermath of a stroke or traumatic brain injury.

I turned off the light, and we recited *Goodnight Moon* together while Katie stroked Eeyore's floppy ears. I said, "I love you" as my hand automatically made the sign.

She signed I love you back as Max, our cat, entered the room. "Good night, Sweetie. Max says good night too."

"Goodnight, Mommy."

She had started using the word Mommy as a name (rather than a noun) a few months earlier. I was still thrilled whenever I heard it.

"Goodbye, Max."

I froze, unsure I'd heard what I thought I heard. Katie had never spontaneously greeted anyone in conjunction with their name. She could say the words, but I needed to coax them out with an indirect prompt.

Max wound around my feet and meowed. Katie giggled. "Good talking, Max."

She'd done it, twice in one night. I wanted to cry and shout and jump on the bed.

So what if it happened a few years late? So what if it wouldn't happen again for months?

Another milestone had been achieved.

Perhaps instead of waiting, I should say keeping the faith. You go a long time without seeing much progress, and just when you are about to lose hope and throw in the towel, something happens to remind you to stay the course, to keep giving the B-12 injections, to keep submitting the endless and redundant paperwork, to keep mixing the supplements when your fingers ache, to keep making calls and fighting for better services.

For example, Katie caught a nasty stomach virus at school and spent the better part of the week lying on the couch, sipping apple juice and watching videos. I asked which video she wanted—*Signing Time* or

Kipper the Dog—and she thought for a moment and said, *"Signing Time*—the purple one."

No prompting, no echoing, no tacking yes at the end of the statement—just an answer to a simple question. I waited four-and-a-half years for her to answer her first question, and four years later, it had finally become second nature.

I wrote it down, so I would remember, but really, I don't need to record such milestones. They are etched in my brain because these are the moments that sustain me.

A few months later, I was sitting on the couch, reading yet another progress report. I wasn't paying much attention to Katie, who was in the kitchen. A voice in my head said, listen. Katie, who has been interested in food since she was a preschooler, was studying photos in a cookbook and talking to herself. "That's soup. Soup is hot. I like chicken tortilla soup. Soup is good. I can make it. I'm stirring soup. I'm stirring tomato soup. Don't slurp your soup. Let's make chicken tortilla soup."

She flipped the page and talked about pumpkin pie. I didn't know she knew what pumpkin pie was. More pages flipped, followed by a long discourse on chocolate cake, then meat, then pasta, then salad with cranberries. It was as if she wanted to say every sentence she could that included the particular food item.

To say I was stunned would be an understatement.

It went on for fifteen minutes, maybe longer.

I listened as the words poured out, barely breathing. Then it hit me. This was it, the moment I'd been waiting for. The words were breaking free, spilling into the kitchen and filling up the room.

They filled me up. Better than any meal.

Joy Comes after the Mourning
MaDonna Maurer

Death. The news of my daughter's diagnosis was like death of a family member.

Matthea was born in China just like her older brother two years before her. In fact, she was born just two doors down from the exact hospital room where he had first entered the world. She was super tiny and had the cutest little kitten-like cry that sounded just like a kitten. Later we would find out that this tiny cat-like cry would be the name of her diagnosis in French, Cri-du-Chat Syndrome.

Unlike her brother, though, she just didn't seem to follow the milestones that all the parenting books had listed. She could not keep her food down. Her spit-ups seemed more like "Old Faithful" than the normal baby spit-ups. She seemed to be sick every few months and wheezed most of the time. At six months of age, I began to worry because she was rolling over but not sitting up. At seven months, she was hospitalized for severe pneumonia.

We did not live in the city where the kids were born. This hospital was different. It wasn't as new and as up-to-date as the hospital in Beijing. The medical equipment looked much older. The pea-green paint cracked and peeled off onto the gray tiled floor. Her room had six beds; four of them with children that had infectious lung diseases. At least her bed sheets seemed clean. Next to that was a tall green oxygen tank with a hose and mask attached. Missing were all the monitors to check her heart rate, oxygen levels, and other vital signs. I remember glancing at my husband whose face reflected my own doubts and fears.

We were instructed to give her oxygen whenever we felt she needed it. At this point, we called our medical insurance company. It was already late at night, but we finally got through to them. We wanted our daughter to be evacuated to a hospital in Beijing. Forty-eight long hours and many phone calls later, we boarded a private plane with a doctor and a nurse who escorted us all the way to Beijing. Doubt and fear were replaced with relief and peace.

It was in Beijing that the pediatrician informed us that her constant sickness was not normal. More testing would be needed to determine the exact cause of her many lung infections. These tests would need to be done in the US.

It was at this point that I was challenged with the thought that maybe this daughter that lay so peacefully in her hospital bed would not be like the daughter I had dreamed of having. She may never walk. She may never play soccer. She may never get married. She may only live a few years. The image of the daughter that I had dreamed of had begun to die.

After another medical evacuation, we arrived in the US fighting jet lag, I drove to the hospital twice a week—two hours one way. It was tiring, but God spoke to me very clearly during that time through encouraging songs on the radio, time with my mother, and even through a surprise visit from some close college friends.

A month and a half later, while waiting in the doctor's office, the pediatrician walked in and told me that he had some good news. My heart jumped with joy and then immediately sunk—good news to a doctor means a diagnosis. I squeezed Matthea a little tighter as we sat down. He began to tell me what my heart was so afraid to hear: my ten-month old daughter was mentally and physically handicapped.

The daughter of my dreams died that day.

She didn't physically die, but everything I had ever thought and imagined about her died. As I explained the diagnosis to my husband, still on the other side of the world, reality sank in and the tears flowed. Fear replaced the uncertainty. Fear of her inabilities, fear of surgery for a feeding tube, fear that we'd have to leave our home in China. Fear tried to strangle me.

I filled my days researching information about this syndrome. I wanted to find the "how to" parent guide for kids with special needs. I wanted the checklist of milestones to help me gauge what we could expect. I found nothing like that, but I did find a support group. That small glimmer of hope encouraged me through those next few weeks.

I was still worried that we'd have to move to the US to take care of Matthea's needs, which would lead to more loss. Loss of friends, since moving away would mean not seeing some of them again. My husband and I consulted therapists, doctors, and surgeons about whether to move back to the US or not. Each one told us without any hesitation to go back to China. The first good news in months, it seemed.

That was nine years ago. We are still living overseas, but no longer in China. I still have moments of grief, and I'm told that parenting a child with special needs stays difficult. It doesn't just "go away." I have found that to be true. Grief finds me at odd places. It finds me at the park where I see girls playing and laughing together while my daughter stumbles up the stairs to go down the slide. Grief finds me in the hospital holding the results from yet another developmental testing, and I see she isn't mentally where I thought she was. And grief brings tears to my eyes when party invitations are passed out, and she didn't get one. Grief reminds me that she doesn't have friends her age. She doesn't seem to notice, but I do. I hurt.

Through all the grief and mourning, joy does come. It always does. It comes with a kiss and a hug. Joy comes with each new word she speaks. It comes when she dresses up in her cowboy hat, boots, and comes out swinging her pretend lasso. Joy comes from watching her love life in the way I sometimes wish I could.

Yes, joy does come after the mourning. It does for me. It will for you, too. Just wait and watch for it.

Acts of Silence

Emily Klein

"Red. Red. Red." I say everything to Joy in three's these days. Then I stare at her lips. They are full and pink and—still. I place the red marker into her art box.

"Up. Up. Up." I speak in triplicate again while I continue to stare at my three-year-old's cupid's bow. I wait for the slightest flicker of movement, proof of a connection between the motor center in her brain and her mouth.

"Yes. Yes. Yes." Her silence stings my ears. The unanswered questions nip at my heart. *Why can't she sit, stand, walk or be nourished without her feeding tube? What can she see?* The doctors' answers—ear piercing silence. Seven months ago, this mystery diagnosis also stole her words. She didn't have many, a handful maybe, "Mama," "Dada," "good girl." They all sounded beautiful.

Joy squirms in my lap. She arches her back to protest the futility of my exercise. I readjust her legs the way her Occupational Therapist showed me with her ankles, knees, and hips all at ninety-degree angles and her feet planted firmly on the floor. My body is her chair.

"Baah—Bah—Baah." I try a sing-song approach. She smiles, exposing an uneven row of baby teeth.

"Can you say, baah-bah-baah?" Joy kicks her feet out in front of her and thrusts her hips forward until she slides down my lap onto the floor. Her back rests against her tan, shag carpet. I brush a dark curl from her eyes.

*

Two teenaged girls and a boy sit shoulder to shoulder on a bench in my friend's backyard. A fire pit crackles and pops in front of them. Remnants of barbeque chicken litter the plates by their bare feet.

I see only their backs and the faces of their phones—all aglow and buzzing.

The teens hold their phones close to their eyes, elbows sealed to their waists, backs slightly rounded. Their thumbs dance frantically around their keypads. They pause briefly—as if taking a breath in a monologue—before continuing.

The boy laughs. The girl to his right stops texting and peers over at his screen. They look at each other and smile. She swings her leg, narrowly missing the plates.

His phone nags at him with a low hum. They return to their silent conversations.

*

My fingers are poised above the keyboard, ready to pounce at my brain's command. I fumble for the right words. I type and delete. Start and stop. My fingers move in fits and bursts until I rest my wrists down on my desk in defeat. I lay my head back on my chair and look up at the ceiling as if in prayer. My fingers still. The silence mocks me and snuffs out my voice.

*

I pile Joy's body into my lap. "Dada. Dada. Dada."

She looks away.

The quiet fills with memories of her voice. It was sweet, yet firm—a child who knows what she wants. That was before the silence crept in between us, a force holding us apart.

Joy pulls her Elmo doll onto her lap. She tugs and twists his furry, red paws until she hits the button. "Elmo loves you." *The doll speaks!* I toss Elmo aside.

"Mama. Can you say, Mama?"

Joy shakes her head, slow, small movements from side to side.

"That's okay," I say. Guilt spreads through my body like a cancer. I pull her to me, feeling her warmth against my breastbone. "You don't have to say it."

I kiss the smooth skin on her forehead. "Kiss." From habit, the word tumbles out of my mouth.

Mwah. Joy's lips pucker and push forward against the air.

"Thank you for the kiss, Joy." I smell the sweet scent of her baby shampoo and murmur into her ear, "Mama loves your kisses."

*

Marcel Mangel was born on March 22, 1923 in Strasbourg, France. He later changed his name and joined the French Resistance during the German occupation. During this time, he worked to save

214

children from the concentration camps. His first pantomime performances were for these children to keep them quiet while they travelled. Wrapped in silence, the children escaped to Switzerland.

He later became one of the world's most treasured artists. Performance halls rumbled with laughter. Sobs also echoed through his theaters; no one could escape the power of his silent personas. Hoards of people collected in movie theaters, huddled around television sets and stuffed into theaters to connect to his genius.

Marcel Marceau left a loud and brilliant mark on the world. His legacy?

"L'art du silence."

*

We step inside the elevator after Joy's neurology appointment. We are alone. My husband hits the button for the main floor, and I position Joy's stroller against the opposite wall. Without speaking, we start the same conversation we have after every doctor's appointment. We no longer need words.

We look at each other. I shake my head and think, *How can all of her test results be normal?*

My husband shrugs. His silence says, *There are no answers. We'll just care for Joy as best as we can.*

I turn away. My lips tighten. My husband moves to me and places his hand on my shoulder. A silent prayer floats between us.

*

I lay Joy down on her blanket and turn on Elmo Radio.

The silence shatters.

I lay next to her and blow a quick breathe against her neck. She raises her hands to my face and laughs, a deep belly laugh that rocks her whole body.

"More?" I ask.

She grins and raises her chin to expose her neck. I blow again, and she squeals in delight.

I scoop her up into my arms and dance around the room. She wraps her small hands around my arms and pulls me tight to her. Our bodies surrender into each other. She nuzzles her head into my chest; her breath resonates a steady rhythm against my heart. Hush. Hush. Hush.

215

Music To My Ears
Tina Traster

There we were, on our winter break vacation, driving to our hotel after a day of skiing in the Canadian Laurentians.

"I miss my violin," Julia sighed, dreamily gazing out at the frozen tundra, not really talking to either my husband or I. Just thinking out loud.

"Really?" I said, whipping my head around to the back seat.

"Yeah, I should have brought it with me," she lamented. "I miss it."

A smile spread across my face. Angels were singing. Julia's words were nothing less than music to my ears.

Julia is good at violin and getting better all the time. Is she destined for Lincoln Center? I doubt it. That's not the point. The fact that she was missing her violin was not about future musical accomplishment. That she was "missing" something was what made this the screech-on-the-brakes moment. It's not like Julia to make a deep attachment or commitment to something, to anything. She's innately intelligent, so she pretty much gallops by at whatever she does or has to do.

But showing passion, well, this was new.

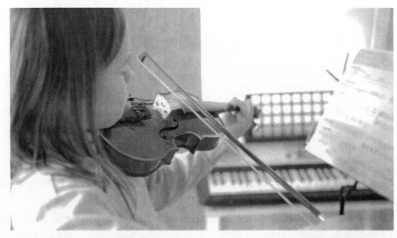

Olga Loginova

216

Julia uttered this comment on practically her tenth Gotcha anniversary. She was eight months old when we adopted her from Siberia a decade ago. Though she was young, Julia had trouble attaching to anyone—or anything—from the moment we brought her home. She never laid claim to a teddy bear or a favorite blanket or toy. She didn't attach to me, my husband, or to other caretakers. She never made a good friend. She was like a drifter, taking what she needed, passing through. When we found a name for this—Reactive Attachment Disorder—we made it our life's work to pull Julia out of her dark tunnel. It took years, and it's never the kind of thing that's completely healed. By the time she was four, we fully understood the syndrome, which is caused by early separation from a birth mother. Babies who don't get the nurture and love they deserve subconsciously learn it's better not to attach to anyone or anything because everything in life, especially love, is ephemeral. A harsh lesson for an infant.

Still, that is what they learn, and these children have a crafty way of keeping their distance and making sure nothing matters too much. It reminds you of someone who's been burned by divorce and decides to close her heart.

At ten, Julia is fully attached to my husband and me. We are a solid forever family, the three of us. But our daughter is still reticent about investing her passion elsewhere. There are no posters of Justin Bieber in her room. No friend from school she calls her BFF. No one thing that really, really matters.

Except maybe her violin?

She took it up in fourth grade in elementary school. She didn't show any particular talent or interest in the instrument. She never practiced at home, but she coasted in the year-end performance. I thought that was the end of that. Then she went to a sleep-away camp for the performing arts. I had been expecting her to be in one of the theatrical shows, but when we got there on visiting day, she played violin in a strings concert. A music teacher had obviously found and mentored her.

When she returned home, I hired a private music teacher. Magical things happened. Julia loves Karen. Karen adores Julia. Julia is getting real good on the violin. She practices every day for thirty minutes. She shows commitment. Passion, even. Music has led her to some part of herself that has cracked open resistance to taking chances and loving something.

A week ago, I told Julia we were going to her Grandmother's for Passover. Grandma was expecting fifteen people.

"Can I bring my violin and play it for everyone?" she asked.

"Please do," I replied.

My Daughter Sings
Dee Thompson

My daughter's voice seeps out from underneath her door,

And soars
Through the dark air of the upper hall
Pure and clear as Joni Mitchell's
Melody threading about
Like beating butterfly wings—
She sings.

My daughter has an auditory processing disorder.
Her brain
Doesn't always correctly comprehend.

Yet she sings.
The radio balanced on her chest, her iPod synced—
She has no idea about singing on key,
Nor does she care.
When I try to teach her, she resists me.
So my years of vocal training, you see,
We cannot share.
Despite her handicap, despite others' disdain,
My daughter sings.
I have never heard anything quite so beautiful.
For a few minutes I forget to be afraid for her.

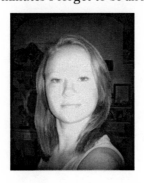

Writing
Prompts

"I know we will have bumps in the road, we already have,
but I know now that I can handle them, maybe not always
with the exact grace I'd like, but we will make it
through…with love and joy."
—Stephanie A. Sumulong

Writing Prompts

Below find writing prompts inspired by the pieces in this collection and from Lyn's work with mothers of children with special needs in the greater Indianapolis community.

We share these prompts in the hope that you too will be inspired to write. Write using whatever genre you want: a narrative, a blog, a poem, a song, a visual. Just write.

Write to describe, write to be heard, write to heal.

In fact, we invite you to join us at
motheringkidswithspecialneeds.wordpress.com
for more great writing and conversation.

Warm Up

- Describe a morning, an event, a quality, or a conversation you want to remember about your child.
- How is your child powerful? Powerless?
- Do you ever feel powerful or powerless?
- What do you want more than anything else for your child?

Digging Deep

- On a good day, I will...
- On a good day, my child will...
- On a bad day, I will...
- On a bad day, my child will...
- Down deep I wish people knew...
- Before my child was born, I...
- After my child was born, I...
- I dream of...

- I am terrified of…
- I have learned to accept…
- I have not learned to accept…
- I have forgiven…

Exploring Environments: Focus on Details, Details, Details

- Take us to that moment when you knew or learned of your child's diagnosis.
- Share a moment of extreme grief. Take us there.
- Share a moment of pure joy. Take us there.
- The most beautiful sound my child makes is…
- The most heartbreaking sound my child makes is…
- Tell us about your day.
- Where do you and your child feel most at peace?

Starting Conversations

- My child is not the problem, but let me tell you what is…
- When you see my child, it's okay to _____, but it's *not* okay to _____.
- Sometimes, we appreciate, even *need*, official jargon and terms, labels and lexes. Other times we prefer euphemisms and cover ups. When you see my child, I want you to use _____. Here's why…
- Sometimes it sucks being a mom to a child with special needs. Here's why…
- Sometimes it's pure joy being a mom to a child with special needs. Here's why…

Using Other Writers as Springboards for Writing and Conversation

- Read "Monday Coffee" by Jo Pelishek. Describe a time when you ached to be selfish, but weren't.

- Read "Melting Clocks" by Anna Yarrow. When do you feel inadequate?

- Read "Torso of Clay" by Christy Spaulding Boyer or "Fragments of the First Five Days" by Jane Dwyer. Do you ever feel like you recollect your life in fragments? What are some of the sharpest fragments your can remember?

- Read "Stopped Holding my Breath" by Carmen Iwaszczenko. What in your life makes you angry?

- Read "My Supposed Life" by Alison Auerbach. Who is your "other you"? Write your "other biography."

- Read "Whatever it Takes" by Claudia Malcrida or "Stopped Holding my Breath" by Carmen Iwaszczenko. Have you ever had to work up the courage to say "no?" Or, do you ever find yourself frantically searching for an answer or something that you just cannot locate?

- Read "When Life Gave Me Lemons, A Pie Was My Weapon" by Julie Mairano. What do you do when you're frustrated? Explore, "When life gives me lemons, I…"

- Read "I Was a Knucklehead" by Heather Kim Lanier. Consider when you've been a knucklehead. Begin, "I used to think _____ about children with special needs."

Contributors

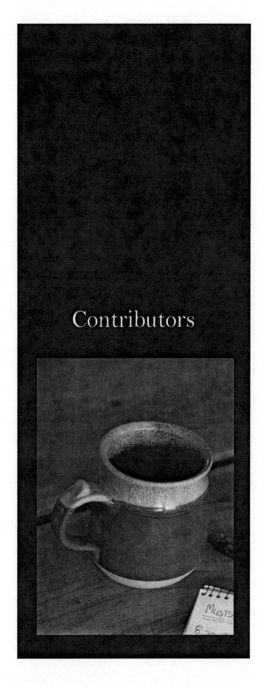

Special parents aren't chosen, they're made.

--Ann Bremer

Contributors

Stacey Anderson is a thirty-something mom of a chubby Chihuahua, Olive, and two boys— Trent Nathaniel (13) and Chase Allen (3). Embracing life as a solo parent, life took an unexpected turn in 2010 when Chase was born with Special Needs. Besides having a fondness for small coffee shops and thrift stores, Stacey adores writing. She shares her journey and newfound strength through online articles, her blog *Solo with Stacey*, and Disability Advocacy for the state of Missouri.

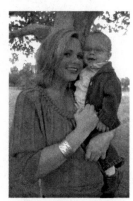

Amanda Apgar lives in Los Angeles with her partner and their daughter, Jane. She is a graduate student in the Department of Gender Studies at University of California, Los Angeles, where she is studying theories of gender and nationalism. Amanda has been blogging for over two years about the ups-and-downs of parenting Jane at
www.positivelyjane.blogspot.com.
This is her first publication.

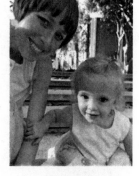

Alison Auerbach is a mom of an awesome autistic son, writer, wife of an extremely patient emergency physician, organization freak, and social worker. She received her BA from Amherst College, MA, and her MSS from the Bryn Mawr Graduate School of Social Work and Social Research, PA. Alison is also the founder of Oxygen MASK (Moms Achieving with Special-needs Kids) and of Ask Me, a supportive consulting service for families of children with special needs.

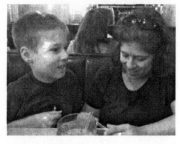

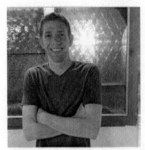

Michael Baumann is a writer, a performer, a musician, a middle child, and a teaching assistant at Ohio University. Building upon a foundation of undergraduate tutoring, public performance poetry, and memoir writing projects with the Indiana Writers' Center, Michael aspires to teach writing and identity rhetorics in the college classroom. He believes that language is powerful, empowering, and messy and that everyone has the aptitude and the license to use it; but not everyone knows it, so his task is to help with that.

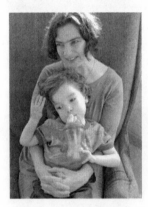

Sally Bittner Bonn is currently working on a book-length memoir about the joys and challenges of raising a son with a physical disability. Her poetry has appeared in *Don't Blame the Ugly Mug*, *Women. Period.*, and *Lake Affect*, among others. She works as the Director of Youth Education at Writers & Books, where she also teaches creative writing. She lives with her husband and son in Rochester, NY. Visit her family's website and blog here: www.oscar-go.org.

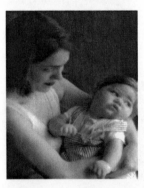

Christy Spaulding Boyer graduated from Anderson University with a BA in Graphic Design. After graduating, she focused on caring for her son, Clay, who needed complete care, alongside his two younger brothers. Clay lived fourteen intense, beautiful years until his death in 2011. Christy is a freelance painter and illustrator. Writing is something she has always done beside her visual work, which is highly influenced by literature. Learn more about Christy at www.christyboyerart.com

Ann Bremer has degrees from Gustavus Adolphus College and the University of Minnesota. She was a contributor to the book *Gifts: Mothers Reflect on How Children with Down Syndrome Enrich Their Lives* She's on the board of directors of KidsCan of Minnesota, an organization that supports families of kids with cancer in Minnesota. She's a wife, stay-at-home-mom, and an aspiring novelist. Her son, John, has Down syndrome and is the fourth of six children. In her free time, she eats squares of dark chocolate.

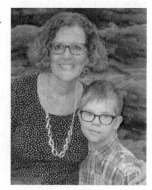

Barbara Crooker's books of poetry are *Radiance*, winner of the Word Press First Book Award and finalist for the Paterson Poetry Prize; *Line Dance*, winner of the Paterson Award for Literary Excellence; *More*; and *Gold*. She was a finalist for the 2012 Pablo Neruda Poetry Prize, and her work appears in *The Bedford Introduction to Literature*. Barbara is the mother of a 29-year-old son with autism who lives with her at home. Learn more at www.barbaracrooker.com.

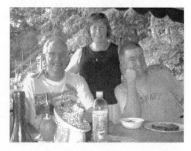

Linda Davis' work has been published in *The Literary Review*, *Gemini Magazine* and, forthcoming, in *Tattoo Highway*. She worked with Antonya Nelson at Bread Loaf and Brad Kessler at Antioch University where she received her MFA. Prior to that, she was story editor at Wild-wood Enterprises, Robert Redford's company, and worked in New York at *Harper's Magazine*. She lives in Santa Monica with her husband and three children. As the mother of a 16-year-old boy with autism, she feels as though she has a degree in Autism, as well.

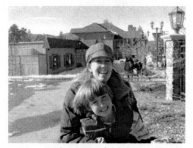

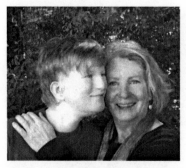

Jane Dwyer is the mother of two children, Amy and Sage, who remain her best teachers. She lives close to the Olympic Mountains where she hikes and plays. She is an artist, gardener, and is working on a memoir about her son, Sage.

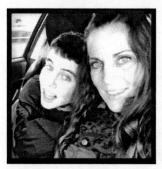

Kimberly Escamilla's recent work has appeared or is forthcoming in *Red Wheelbarrow, Voices of Hellenism, Plath Profiles, Huffington Post, 5AM, DMQ Review,* and *My Baby Rides the Short Bus* anthology. She has taught college-level writing and literature in the San Francisco Bay Area for 19 years and is the Director of The International Poetry Library of San Francisco. Kimberly lives on the coast, a few miles north Half Moon Bay, CA with her husband Michael and sons Harrison and Lazlo.

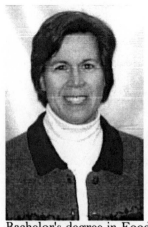

Margaret Hentz has been delivering back-of-the book subject and name indexes for publishers, packagers, and authors for more than 25 years covering a wide range of subjects including chemistry, physics, biology, and nutrition, legal, psychology, history, religion, music, aviation, and theatre. Margaret has more than 25 years of information management experience working as a Research Librarian at Research and Development (R&D) libraries in various Fortune 500 corporations. She has a Bachelor's degree in Food Science with a minor in Chemistry, Masters in Library Science (M.L.S.) and a Doctorate in Library and Information Science (D.S.I.S.).

Carmen Noller Iwaszczenko is a Midwestern genetics laboratory professional, a wife, and a mother of two, including a son with high functioning autism. She is teaching herself to navigate life as a parent of a child with Asperger's as gracefully as possible whilst still managing to maintain a backbone. She is family-focused, yet manages to eke out free time for enjoying photography, Rieslings, and any movie or musical starring a certain Hugh Jackman.

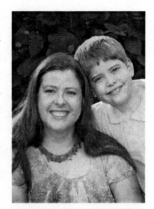

Darolyn "Lyn" Jones is a mom to a son with a disability, a wife, a teacher, a writer, a sister friend, and a social activist. She is an Assistant Professor in the Department of English at Ball State University and the Education Outreach Director of the Indiana Writers Center, where

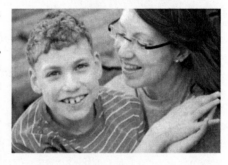

she has facilitated several urban outreach writing programs, including Girls in Prison Speak, Sitting at the Feet of our Elders, Building a Rainbow, Recording War Memories, CityWrite, and Special Needs Moms Write. Lyn is passionate about literacy and has devoted her personal and professional life to teaching and writing with writers both in and out of the classroom. Check out her website, publications, and blog at www.darolynlynjones.com

Suzanne Kamata is an American who lives in Japan with her Japanese husband and their teenaged twins. She is the author of two novels, including most recently, *Gadget Girl: The Art of Being Invisible* (GemmaMedia, 2013), which features a biracial girl with cerebral palsy and a short story

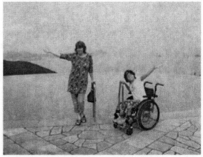

collection. Suzanne is the editor of three anthologies, including *Love You to Pieces: Creative Writers on Raising a Child with Special Needs* (Beacon Press, 2008). Learn more at www.suzannekamata.com.

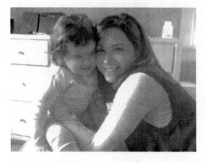

Emily Klein is a writer, wife and mother of two young daughters. When she is not busy with her girls, she spends her time writing about them. Emily also volunteers at her older daughter's school for children with special needs. She writes for *Barista Kids* and has work scheduled for publication in *Literary Mama* and *The Healing Muse*

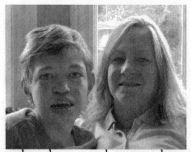

Sharon Hecker Kroll is a wife and mother who lives with her three favorite men: her husband, Tom, and sons Mikey and Matthew. She is grateful to Tom for his infinite love and patience, which makes this journey easier; to Matt, who is a wonderful son and brother and makes her proud every day; and to Mikey, who has Angelman syndrome, and teaches her to enjoy the wonders of each new day. In her spare time, she enjoys read-ing, gardening, walking and playing with the dogs; Sadie and Otis. This is her first publication.

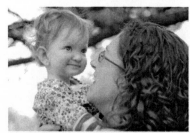

Heather Kirn Lanier is the author of the memoir *Teaching in the Terrordome: Two Years in West Baltimore with Teach For America* (U of Missouri) and the poetry chapbook *The Story You Tell Yourself* (Kent State). Her work has appeared in dozens of places, including *Salon* and *The Sun*. Heather blogs about her daughter at starinhereye.wordpress.com.

Mark Latta directs CityWrite, a city-wide memoir project in Indianapolis. His interest in public literacy and socio–linguistics has led to multiple ethnography and memoir projects centered on human experience through language and shared narratives. He has edited and assisted in the creation of numerous anthologies and is a recipient of the Nuvo Cultural Vision Award and the William H. Plater Civic Engagement Medallion. He 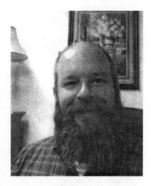 works with the Indiana Writers Center Memoir Project as an instructor and technical editor, and is the Assistant Director of the Marian University Writing Center. More importantly, he has an amazing wife, Martha. They share a home with three dogs, four cats, and a brood of chickens.

Robin LaVoie holds a MA in Public History from Arizona State University, in addition to her more cherished credential of Mom to one quirky, mysterious, and lovable teenaged boy. She splits her time between providing historical research, writing, and editing services and helping her son navigate the world outside of the autism spectrum. Robin hoards spare 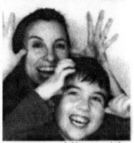 moments to write at stayquirkymyfriends.wordpress.com and lives with her husband and son in Fountain Hills, Arizona.

Leslie Mahoney is a registered nurse currently working for the California Department of Public Health who participates in Medicare inspections of skilled nursing facilities. Her nursing career has included 25 years in intensive care units both as a staff nurse and a director, developing a hospital- 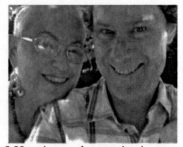 based home health agency, Director of Hospice and a geriatric care manager. Leslie is a single parent of two sons and a joyful grandmother. She is socially and politically active in health care related issues, especially senior care and end of life decisions.

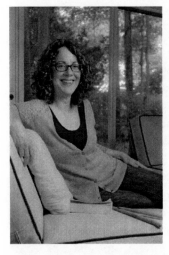

Liz Main frequently writes on topics related to music and popular culture, with several recent essays appearing in *Punchnel's*. Liz's debut novel, *Now That We're Here*, tells the story of an alcoholic mother raising an autistic son in affluent Bergen County, New Jersey. Find out more at www.lizmain.me.

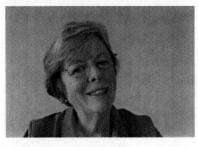

Julie Mairano is a mother, wife, and grandmother of five who hopes to change the world for children like her daughter who was born with Cornelia de Lange syndrome (CdLS). As Executive Director of the CdLS Foundation, she led the organization through a period of substantial growth. Since retirement she has been active as a consultant for Boston nonprofits with ESC of New England and is honored to play a significant role in the creation of a CdLS Center at Children's Hospital of Philadelphia.

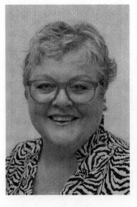

Claudia Malacrida teaches and researches at the University of Lethbridge on Sociology of Disability, Gender and Motherhood. Claudia has published several books on these topics, including "Cold Comfort: Mothers, Professionals and ADHD," "Sociology of the Body," and the forthcoming "A Special Hell: Institutional Life in the Eugenic Years." Her daughter Hilary is now a journeywoman electrician who owns a horse, lives on her own, and is having a great life.

MaDonna Maurer currently lives with her husband and three children in Taiwan, where she assists her husband with Taiwan Sunshine, a nonprofit organization for families of children with special needs. Her passion is teaching third culture kids and writing. She finds time to do both between the endless demands of the household plus all that is en-tailed in raising a child with special needs. She can be found blogging at www.raisingtcks.com.

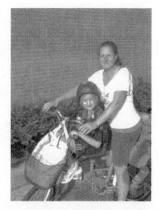

Jennifer Meade is a licensed clinical social worker with a Master's degree in Social Work from the University of Chicago and a BA in Sociology from the University of Illinois. She has dedicated the past 20 years of her life to helping others navigate life's

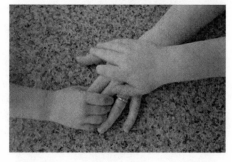

complicated challenges, which still left her largely unprepared to navigate her own. She lives in Chicago with her two beautiful boys and über-cheerleader of a husband. Jennifer currently works for her alma mater preparing the next generation of social workers to help society's most marginalized members. In her rare free moments, she tries to carve out time to pursue her creative passion, writing. Her approach to parenting, and to life in general, is to grade herself on a pass/fail scale.

Brian McGuckin is an award-winning photographer featured in multiple publications. Photography has allowed him to pursue his dream of capturing life from his local home in Indiana to all over the world; from backyards, to red carpets, to NFL football fields. He most enjoys living life with his beautiful wife Rebecca and their four children. Learn more at www.brianmcguckin.com.

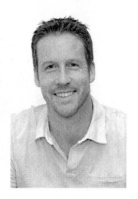

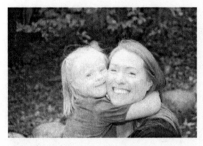

Michele McLaughlin has a BS from North Dakota State University as well as an MBA from European University in Barcelona. Her past adventures include riding a train around Europe, climbing Mt. Kilimanjaro, starting her own business, and even jumping out of an airplane. She is currently enjoying her newest adventure as mom to an amazing daughter who happens to have Down syndrome and an incredible son who happens not to. They live in Minneapolis.

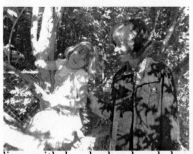

Ellen E. Moore has degrees in creative writing from the University of Wisconsin-Madison (BS) and the University of Alaska Fairbanks (MFA) and in Library Science from Indiana University (MLS). She currently works at a public library in Marquette, Michigan where she lives with her husband and daughter. She's published a dozen or so poems in literary journals and one short story. She didn't know a damn thing about autism till 2010, when it became very apparent she'd better learn all she could.

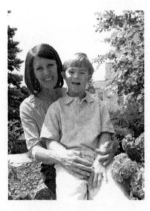

Deborah Leigh Norman grew up in Delaware and later moved to Virginia, Louisiana, and now Indiana. She is enjoying the journey of living in different regions of our country as well as the journey of her heart becoming a mother and then the mother of a child with a disability. Deborah Leigh has a BA and MPA from the University of Delaware. Come share your journey with her at www.departingholland.com.

Michelle Odland has a degree in English from UW Oshkosh in English. She lives in Wisconsin with her husband and their three children. Michelle learned what she needed to know about Down syndrome with the birth of her second child, Nyssa. It is a work in progress. She spends her free time volunteering with Special Olympics and JDRF and learning about life from her children. You can learn more from her at www.mylifewiththree.wordpress.com.

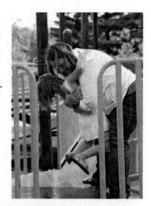

Mary E. Overfield is currently a full-time at-home caregiver for her 16-year-old medically compromised daughter, Megan, who has multiple disabilities, as well as her 17-year-old daughter, Emily. She is married to Dane and they all live in Rochester, NY. Mary has a BS in Accounting from Gannon University in Erie, PA

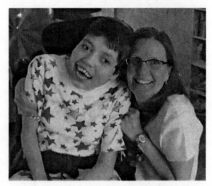

and she enjoys writing about being a "special needs mom." This is her first submission of a literary piece for publication, and Mary is excited to be a part of the Mother's Anthology Project.

Jamie Pacton lives, teaches, and writes near the shores of Lake Michigan in Milwaukee. She's a Columnist and Contributing Editor at the *Autism and Aspergers Digest* and her work has appeared in *The Writer, Cricket, Parents,* and many other publications. When she's not grading papers or at her

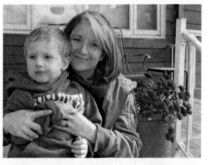

computer working on her YA novel, she's usually at the zoo, park, pool, or art museum with her two young sons (one of whom has autism, and both of whom are magnificent). You can learn more about Jamie at her blog, www.jamiepacton.com.

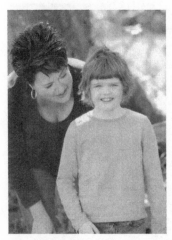

Cynthia J. Patton is a special needs attorney and founder of the non-profit organization, Autism A to Z. Her award-winning nonfiction and poetry have appeared in eleven anthologies, including the best-selling *Chicken Soup for the Soul* series, plus numerous print and online publications. In 2012, her story, *Elliott Comes to Play*, was performed on stage. This Northern California native is completing a memoir on her unconventional journey to motherhood. Learn more at http://CynthiaJPatton.com

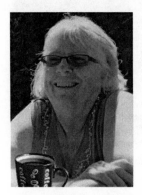

Jo Pelishek draws on her experience of raising five children, three of whom had disabilities. She has a background in journalism with a B.A. from Augsburg College, Minneapolis. Jo has worked as a disability advocate for several years, doing individual as well as systems advocacy. She and her husband live on a lake in northwest Wisconsin. When not working or writing, Jo enjoys time with family and Skyping with her granddaughters in California.

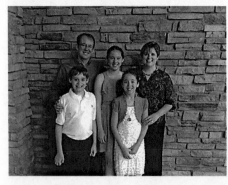

Christina K. Searcy has a BS in computer engineering from the University of Notre Dame. After having an eleven-year full-time internship, she decided to make it official and is currently working on an M.A. in special education and applied behavior analysis with a certificate in autism from Ball State University. She lives in Westfield, Indiana with her three children and husband and works part-time as a behavior therapist, set designer and theater instructor. She has illustrated a children's book and enjoys singing, painting and acting in her free time.

Bridgette Shively lives in Muncie, Indiana. She has her bachelor's degree in Creative Writing, and is currently working towards obtaining her teaching license from Ball State University. Bridgette is a serial hobbyist and enjoys dabbling in various forms of art, including drawing.

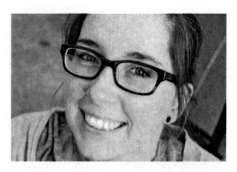

Stephanie Sumulong is mom to a young son with Down syndrome. She is also an online social studies teacher, although she considers working with her son to be her most rewarding teaching "assignment." Stephanie writes a blog, *The Sumulong 3*, chronicling the triumphs and challenges raising

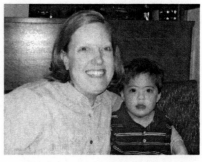

her son and has had several posts featured on other blogs, the *International Down Syndrome Coalition, Down Syndrome Blogs,* and *Down Syndrome Daily.* This is her first formal published work.

Dee Thompson lives in Atlanta and is a freelance writer. She currently writes blogs, books, essays, and the occasional poem. Dee holds an MA in Creative Writing from the University of Tennessee. She is the author of two books, *Adopting Alesia* and *Jack's New Family,* and contributed an essay to *The Divinity of Dogs.* Dee also blogs at *The Crab*

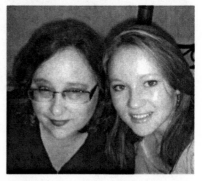

Chronicles, and her professional blog, *The Write Rainmaker.* Dee lives with her son and enjoys gardening, cooking, knitting, reading, and movies.

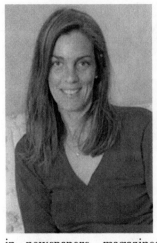

Tina Traster is an adoptive parent of a girl from Siberia and a journalist, columnist and essayist. She is writing a memoir about parenting her daughter, who was eight months old when she was adopted and had attachment issues. Her memoir, *Rescuing Julia Twice*, which will be published by Chicago Review Press (2014), is a story of despair, hope and small miracles. Traster, who is a *New York Post* columnist and a *Huffington Post* and *Daily Beast* blogger, has written several essays about adoption. Her works have appeared in newspapers, magazines, including *Adoptive Families Magazine*, literary journals, several "mommy" blogs, and on NPR. Her essays have been anthologized in literary collections *Living Lessons, Nurturing Paws, Little Blessings* and *Mammas and Pappas.* She is the author of *Burb Appeal Too* and *Hits & Misses: New York Entrepreneurs Reveal Their Strategies.* Traster's website on her adoption story is www.juliaandme.com. She has produced the video "The Kids Are Not Alright," which is on the site. Traster also maintains another website, www.tinatraster.com, where her work is archived.

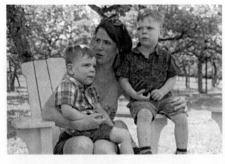

Tracey Trousdell lives on the west coast of Canada with her husband, daughter, and identical twin boys. The twins, born more than three months early, have Cerebral Palsy. A former Project Manager turned stay-at-home mom, Tracey uses her organizational and time management skills to enthusiastically boss her family around. Her blog, www.traceytrousdell.com, is a sometimes funny, sometimes heart-wrenching, all-the-time authentic look at her family living life to the fullest through adversity.

Liz Whiteacre teaches creative writing at Ball State University. Poems about her own experiences with accident and disability have appeared in *Wordgathering, Disability Studies Quarterly, Breath and Shadow,* and other magazines, and her chapbook, *Hit the Ground,* is now available from Finishing Line 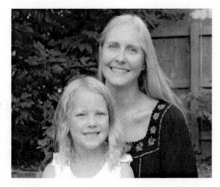 Press. When she's not editing, Liz enjoys going on adventures with her husband and daughter. Learn more at whiteacrehitstheground.wordpress.com.

Anna Yarrow is an introvert who often feels like hiding in a cave. Her daughter, Aria, is an extrovert who calls "Mom!" three hundred times a day. Thankfully, they both love to read. Anna lived overseas for twelve years. She taught typing in Guyana, sang in nightclubs in South Africa, photographed royal weddings and directed art exhibitions in the Sultanate of Oman. This is her first 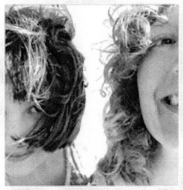 time in print in the USA. Her website is http://www.annayarrow.com.

Aria Eden Mair was born in the Middle East. She is eight years old. She's honored to have poems and an essay about her in this book.

Acknowledgements

We wish to gratefully acknowledge the support of these organization and individuals:

Barbara Shoup, Executive Director of the Indiana Writers Center

Mark Latta, Assistant Director of the Writing Center at Marian University, Technical Editor for INwords Press, and CityWrite Indianapolis Program Director for The Indiana Writers Center

Michael Baumann, Student Intern and Editor for INwords Press

Bridgette Shively, Graphic Artist

Brian McGuckin of Brian McGuckin Photography for cover art.

We wish to thank all of the individual donors who contributed to our Power2Give site and helped make this book possible.

We gratefully acknowledge and thank Chase Bank for matching every contributing dollar from our individual donors.

And thanks to Midwest Orthotics and Technology Center for their financial support and for their support of families who have children with special needs.

We would also like to acknowledge publishers who previously supported writers' work:

> *Literary Mama*, who will publish Emily Klein's "Acts of Silence"
> *Vox Poetica*, who first published Dee Thompson's "My
> Daughter Sings"
> *Adoptive Families Magazine*, who first published Tina Traster's
> "Music to My Ears"

About INwords Publications &
The Indiana Writers Center Memoir Project

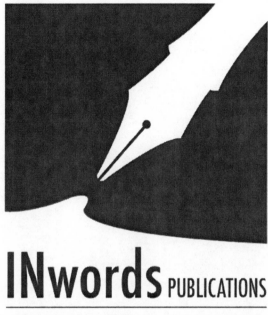

INwords PUBLICATIONS

PRESENTED BY THE INDIANA WRITERS CENTER

INwords Publications is the imprint of the Indiana Writers Center. It publishes books about the writing craft, as well as anthologies produced by its memoir projects.

The IWC believes that everybody has a story worth telling, and its memoir classes and projects are designed to help people of all ages and background to tell theirs, using a curriculum that helps them identify meaningful moments, see them in their mind's eyes, and bring them alive on the page in vivid, compelling scenes.

Memoir Project classes are taught by experienced IWC instructors and, occasionally, by guest teachers who specialize in memoir. Special projects serve particular audiences whose voices are not usually heard, such as senior citizens, veterans, juvenile offenders, and special needs moms. You can learn more about the Memoir Project at http://www.indianawriters.org.

We also invite you to join us online at our blog *Monday Coffee & Other Stories*, www.motheringkidswithdisabilities.wordpress.com.

Index

A

Ableist, 127, 128, 151
Acceptance of special needs child, 156–157
    by friends, 165–169
    by parents upon diagnosis, 3–4, 22–37, 104–111, 112–116, 126–129,
        149–152, 172–174
    by relatives, 43–46, 68–70
    by strangers, 40, 184–187
Accessibility for handicapped persons, 15–21
ADD. *See* Attention deficit disorder (ADD)
ADHD. *See* Attention deficit hyperactivity disorder (ADHD)
Adjusting to living with special needs child, 104–106
Aging out of special needs parents, 62–66
Anxiety over time, 62
Applied behavioral analysis (ABA), 181–812
ASD. *See* Autism spectrum disorder (ASD)
Asperger's syndrome, 11–14
Attachment, lack of, 216–219
Attention deficit disorder (ADD), 91–100
Attention deficit hyperactivity disorder (ADHD), 2
Auditory processing disorder, 219
Autism, 11–14, 25–26, 36–37, 62,124–125, 179–180
    changes in home environment, 29–30
    dealing with medical profession, 31–32
    diagnosing, 28–29
    incidence of, 31
    medication for, 31–32
    negative impact on mother, 33–34
    reaction to by others, 43
    sensory sensitivity, 179–180, 190–196
    sensory underactivity compensation, 34
    with mental retardation, 36–37
Autism spectrum disorder (ASD), 62, 206
Autistic people, employing, 124–125
Autistic savants, 195–196
Avonex, 68–69

B

C

D

E

F

G

H

I

Isolation
of autistic children, 166
of special needs mothers, iii, 53

J

Joint Attention, 181-182
Jobs for autistic people, 124-125
Joy of having special needs child, 170, 175-178, 183–187, 216–218

K

Kingsley, Emily Perl, 156
Kissing, aversion to by autistic children, 179-180
Kyphosis, 51

L

Lears, Jackson, 33
Leukemia, 159
Life sharing for autistic adults, 62
Lingering between life and death, 138-145

M

Marceau, Marcel, 214
Mental retardation 36, 150
Mental retardation with autism, 35-36
Misbehavior *vs.* disability, 45-46
Motivation of autistic children, 48
Multiple sclerosis (MS), 68-71

N

O

P

R

S

What Others Are Saying About Monday Coffee & Other Stories of Mothering Children with Special Needs

"An exceptional compilation of writings. This is very important reading for educators, physicians, therapists and anyone who works with families of children with special needs. It will make us laugh and make us cry. And most importantly, it will open our eyes and help us to understand and support more effectively."

— Dr. Ina Whitman,
Neonatologist,
St. Vincent Women's Hospital

"In Monday Coffee & Other Stories of Mothering Children with Special Needs, the authors deal with severe hardships generated by children who suffer from debilitating conditions that require constant care and a society in general that grows less inclined – or financially able if you prefer political correctness over truth – to help. They all deal with the guilt, frustration, anger, and pain this struggle causes. Each mother has learned to do that in her own way and has become stronger. What these narratives share with us, as readers, is a sense of hope translated into language through the grace of the actions that created the words. Do humanity a favor and contribute to a worthy enterprise by buying this book. Do yourself a favor by reading it."

—Jim McGarrah,
award-winning author of
A Temporary Sort of Peace and Breakfast at Denny's

"'Special parents aren't chosen, they're made' says Ann Bremer in an essay from this remarkable book. Forged is more like it, or annealed perhaps, in a crucible you cannot comprehend unless you, too, have been the parent of a child with Autism, or Down Syndrome, or Cerebral Palsy, or any of the other conditions gathered under the currently-popular sobriquet of 'special needs.' These haunting essays and poems returned me to the early, dark time of my son's birth and diagnosis, before I picked my cautious way, as these authors do, through the ruins of a naïve dream of the perfect, golden family back into gratitude for the families that we have.

On this journey, society fails special moms and their special needs kids. Our friends fail us, and our families, and sometimes our spouses and lovers. Visits and calls dwindle, and when we go out, it is into a world that can be hostile or at best insensitive. People wonder why we kept our child alive or do not have him or her shut away. What is left, but to draw on our own resources and create our own, new ideas of perfection and community? There is no Pollyanna hope in this honest, raw book, but the writing resonates with complex emotions that transcend despair. I came away with empathy and admiration for the fierce faith and fortitude of these mothers, who remind me of those in support groups I joined and founded when my son was in grammar school. While other parents fretted over invitations to parties and college applications, we wondered things like, will my child ever say the word 'Mom'? Who will care for him when I am gone? Who will pay for that? Who will love him? Or, even, will my child still be alive the fall of his or her senior year?

And yet, somehow, we go on. Partly by learning appreciation for the smallest gifts. 'Rather than bemoan that my daughter might not be able to swallow' Heather Kin Lanier says, 'I reveled in the amazement that was swallowing, and humanity's overwhelming adeptness at it. We were geniuses out there! All of us! Swallowing!' We go on by learning to re-frame our visions of perfection. And we go on, too, because we have each other. And we have books like this one, to remind us with power and grace how to endure what we sometimes fear we cannot."

—Rebecca Foust,
award-winning author of
God, Seed, All That Gorgeous Pitiless Song,
and a new manuscript shortlisted for the
Dorset and Kathryn A.Morton prizes

CPSIA information can be obtained at www.ICGtesting.com
Printed in the USA
LVOW13s0508021213

363484LV00002B/5/P